Onward

Jennifer Pien • Lisa Jacobs
Jennifer Soh
Editors

Onward

Narratives at the Heart of Medicine

Springer

Editors
Jennifer Pien
Department of Psychiatry and Behavioral Sciences
Stanford University School of Medicine
Stanford, CA, USA

Lisa Jacobs
Department of Psychiatry and Behavioral Sciences
Stanford University School of Medicine
Stanford, CA, USA

Jennifer Soh
Stanford University
Stanford, CA, USA

Associate Editor
Ray Zhang
Columbia University
New York, NY, USA

ISBN 978-3-032-15775-1 ISBN 978-3-032-15776-8 (eBook)
https://doi.org/10.1007/978-3-032-15776-8

This Springer imprint is published by the registered company Springer Nature Switzerland AG
The registered company address is: Gewerbestrasse 11, 6330 Cham, Switzerland

Foreword

Patients effuse story. Etched between the lines of their medical histories, their chronicles reflect the extraordinary experiences that define a life. Each story is woven with threads of victories and troubles, decorated with snapshots of glee and gloom.

From the bustling halls of the hospital to the quiet single-shingle office, the observant physician witnesses the intimacies of lives, of tragedies, of help, of recovery, of hope, of loss. Detecting and appreciating these narratives can be as crucial to the practice of medicine as deciphering clinical data.

Being busy, physicians typically don't find the time to tap out their yarns, even though many are spellbinding. The physician may mention a story to a colleague over coffee, or a spouse over dinner, but then the memory fades into the mist.

But some doctors put the work into sharing. They realize their experiences make for page-turning tales that those outside the corridors of medicine find miraculous, tear-jerking, heart-rending, inspiring, or insightful. And those physicians will sometimes put down their stethoscope to pick up their pen—among them William Carlos Williams, Sir Arthur Conan Doyle, Michael Crichton, Robin Cook, Oliver Sacks, Khaled Hosseini, Atul Gawande, Abraham Verghese, Anton Chekhov, Siddhartha Mukherjee, Oliver Wendell Holmes Sr., Paul Kalanithi, and hundreds more.

Among these physician-writers, I had the pleasure to know one personally. We were in the same department at the Stanford University School of Medicine, and soon after arriving, I had the pleasure of meeting Dr. Hans Steiner, one of the most ebullient people I've known. I was amazed when I learned he was over 70 years old: he had the energy and enthusiasm of someone half his age.

Hans was born a year after the end of World War II in Vienna, Austria. He became the first in his family to attend university, and he then graduated from the University of Vienna as a doctor of medicine. After residencies, he joined the Stanford School of Medicine faculty in 1981, where he authored or edited an enormous number of articles, reviews, and books. He was awarded Lifetime Distinguished Fellow by the American Psychiatric Association.

In his last years, Steiner was working on his second novel, the first having been written when he was a medical student.

Recognizing the power of literature and seeing the lack of an organization to speed this along, Hans did what any super-enthusiastic person does: he was struck with the sudden idea to start a group. In 2008, he formed *Pegasus Physician Writers* at Stanford, along with Audrey Shafer, MD (Anesthesia), Irvin Yalom, MD (Psychiatry), and Larry Zaroff, MD, PhD (Cardiac Surgery).

The group was founded for physicians who loved creative writing. It soon budded off a medical literary journal, *The Pegasus Review*, under the wing of Jennifer Pien, MD (Psychiatry).

Hans spread the word throughout the medical school for years, pulling together anyone—from students to retired faculty—who wanted to write about medicine.

As of this writing, *Pegasus Physician Writers* has over 220 members from all branches of medicine, and collectively they've published almost 100 books over the past decade. Members write poetry, fiction, fictionalized memoirs, op-ed pieces, and educational texts. Why? The stated goal is to broaden public understanding of the science and art of medicine. The private reason is because they love to commit their world on the page.

The mission goes the other way as well: bringing the insights of the humanities to the practice of medicine. In this way, they can educate medical students and young physicians in the humanistic dimensions of medical practice, and to celebrate the lives of patients through their writing.

This book is a collection of essays, stories, and poems from those who took Hans up on his big idea. The authors all combined time at the bedside with time at the keyboard. The following pages contain the gems of those with medical training who had something to report: something that would keep them up late into the night, tap-tapping on a laptop while their colleagues watched TV or dozed off.

Just as they were the lucky recipients of Hans' enthusiasm, we are the lucky readers of their offerings.

Department of Psychiatry
Stanford University School of Medicine
Stanford, CA, USA
October 2023

David Eagleman

Contents

Contributors

Benjamin Amendolara Los Angeles County Department of Mental Health, Homeless Outreach & Mobile Engagement (HOME) Program, Los Angeles, CA, USA

Steve Asch Department of Medicine, Stanford University School of Medicine, Palo Alto, CA, USA

Alexandra Belardo-DeFelice Department of Psychiatry and Behavioral Sciences, Tulane University, New Orleans, LA, USA

Matthew Bucknor Department of Radiology and Biomedical Imaging, University of California, San Francisco, San Francisco, CA, USA

Arjun S. Byju Department of Radiology, University of California Davis, Medical Center, Sacramento, CA, USA

Megan Campany Division of Cardiothoracic Surgery, Department of Surgery, University of North Carolina at Chapel Hill, Chapel Hill, NC, USA

Hannah Decker Department of Surgery, University of California San Francisco, San Francisco, CA, USA

Rebecca Grossman-Kahn Psychiatry, HealthPartners, St Paul, MN, USA

Rachel H. Han Psychiatry, Walter Reed National Military Medical Center, Bethesda, MD, USA

Lisa Jacobs Department of Psychiatry and Behavioral Sciences, Stanford University School of Medicine, Stanford, CA, USA

Allison Neeson Department of Pediatrics, Children's Hospital of Philadelphia, Philadelphia, PA, USA

Jennifer Pien Department of Psychiatry and Behavioral Sciences, Stanford University School of Medicine, Stanford, CA, USA

Ava Satnick Stanford University School of Medicine, Stanford, CA, USA

Brian Smith Department of Medicine, Stanford University School of Medicine, Stanford, CA, USA

Jennifer Soh Stanford University, Stanford, USA

Hans Steiner Department of Psychiatry and Behavioral Sciences, Stanford University School of Medicine, Stanford, CA, USA

Richard Wu Psychiatry and Behavioral Sciences, Johns Hopkins Hospital, Baltimore, MD, USA

1 Code

Benjamin Amendolara

I was in the ER doc box with the other residents when the charge nurse stuck her head in and said a CPR patient was on the way. A 33-year-old woman, compressions started 10 minutes after she was found.

The senior resident hustled out of the room. I followed. This was all new to me. I had only ever participated in codes on mannequins whose ribs didn't crack when you forced the whole weight of your upper body down on their chests.

People in the ER started moving. Really moving. Like a storm was coming, and we were boarding up windows. Clear the halls! Someone yelled. Guided by some unspoken choreography, a whole team of residents, nurses, respiratory therapists, pharmacists, and ER techs assembled at the anticipated bedside. I squeezed into the room and looked at others for cues on what to do. I breathed.

This was happening.

People in the hallway pressed themselves to the wall as paramedics propelled the gurney-strapped patient to the room. They parked the gurney next to the bed, said one, two, three, and heaved her over. Shears tore through her clothes, and suddenly she was naked.

B. Amendolara (✉)
Los Angeles County Department of Mental Health, Homeless Outreach & Mobile Engagement (HOME) Program, Los Angeles, CA, USA

J. Pien et al. (eds.), *Onward*,
https://doi.org/10.1007/978-3-032-15776-8_1

Deft hands connected the ECG leads, O_2 sat reader, compression monitor, and blood pressure cuff. The nurse couldn't get an IV in, so someone jammed an intraosseous line into her tibia.

A resident hopped up onto a stool and began compressions, throwing his body weight into every one. The intern bag-ventilated. The nurse drew up epinephrine. People did what they were supposed to do.

After 2 minutes, the senior resident told me to take over compressions. I stepped onto the stool, clasped my hands onto the compression monitor over her sternum, and began.

I watched the monitor, focused on keeping the numbers from screaming red. My arms burned faster than I thought they would. Forty seconds, said the senior resident. I thought he had miscounted. I kept going.

When 2 minutes was up, the other resident jumped back on. I stood to the side, huffing, my fingers on the patient's pulse. As my breath calmed and the world seemed to rearrange itself around me, I saw her, the patient, as if for the first time.

Shawna. She was Black, obese, and 33. Overdose? Someone asked. Her skin sloshed out in all directions. Home-done tattoos (you could tell by the faded, imprecise ink) all over. "Pain is inevitable" on her forearm. "Faith" on her other forearm. "Stay alive" on the inside of her index finger. There was some Runic design of scars on her thigh that I couldn't decipher. Branding? The senior resident called out for 2 minutes. I took over.

This time I watched her face. Her head jostled like a doll's. Her eyes bulged, the vasculature bloody and swollen, lids open, staring at nothing. Vomit caked around her lips. A little bit shot out with every compression, with every pump of the bag. There was vomit in her hair, on her shoulders, on my gloves. Her hair had recently been straightened. Her skin bloomed darkly just below where I was slamming into her chest. A rib cracked. I was getting tired. Two minutes. I hopped down.

I clamped my fingers on where her pulse should have been and turned my attention back to the design on her thigh. It hit me. These were cuts, deeper and wider than I had ever seen. They were on her wrists too, her upper arms, her belly, her feet.

Scattered among them were deep, jagged caverns. Gouges, burns. Like she'd been tortured. Her arm dangled off the bed. I held it back to her side.

Let's do one more round, then call it, said the senior.

Somehow, we achieved ROSC. A thready pulse reawakened in her femoral artery. I closed my eyes and separated the blood slamming through my fingertips from hers.

It's there, I said.

We provided supportive care for the next 10 minutes, then the gloves came off, PPE ripped away, pages responded to. The sounds of the ER crept back in, fully alive. If someone had been on a break, they might not have noticed anything had happened at all.

It was just me and the ER tech in the room amidst the remains: vomit-crusted chucks, used-up syringes, torn packages, sodden sheets. I looked over her body. I made note of her scars, tattoos, hair, nails, birthmarks, and piercings. As though I were wading through her life. It got hard to breathe. Pressure built behind my eyes, a deep, unstoppable pressure like when you are aware of some terrible inevitability.

I snuck off to the empty resident lounge. In the sanctity of a big open room with posters urging masks, pictures of happy residents, and flyers for the union, I cried. It was one of the only times in my adult life I did. It felt uncomfortable. I felt weak, exposed.

Back in the doc box, I overheard that her EEG showed brain death. The news didn't hit me. By that point, I was already exhausted. I sleepwalked through the rest of my shift and drove home. I avoided emails, phone calls, texts—anything that reminded me that life could go on normally. I slept a restless sleep. Vague nightmares about research and evaluations, none of Shawna. But when I woke, her face, lifeless but also full of life, or the history of life, hovered over everything like a silk screen.

I didn't know who she was. Her scars told me she was deeply unhappy, or at least lost. Abused. Trapped. Scared. Her tattoos suggested sex trafficking. A victim of a cruel society. Cruel people. Or maybe it wasn't any of that.

I just didn't know.

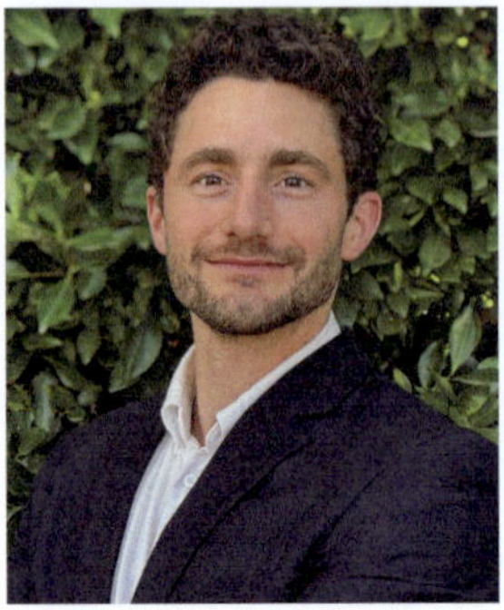

Benjamin Amendolara, MD is a Los Angeles psychiatrist who completed UCLA School of Medicine and UCSD residency. He works with unhoused patients, particularly those with psychotic disorders, while running a private practice. He recently walked the Camino in France and enjoys sculpting, boxing, and tending his garden alongside his two cats.

Socks

2

Alexandra Belardo-DeFelice

On hospital day 1, I nearly missed him. The techs were loading him onto the stretcher so he could go get an abdominal ultrasound— "Please," I asked them, "Can I have just a few minutes? I'll be quick."

I was begging. I had just switched from Team A to Team Heart, and this was my first new patient. Not only was this a new attending, but also a new senior and new interns. I had to do well. I had to make a good impression, even though I was pretty sure, 3 weeks into this 6-week rotation, that IM was not exactly my strong suit.

On IM, the only thing I ever knew for sure was that I didn't know what I was doing.

The techs granted my request, and I knelt down so I was at the patient's level. The first thing I noticed was his dramatically increased work of breathing, which was expected. I introduced myself and asked how he was doing, even though I could have guessed. I rushed through the review of systems and found myself lingering on the social history—the worst of my perpetual faults, the stumbling block in my approach that I can't seem to skip over.

A. Belardo-DeFelice (✉)
Department of Psychiatry and Behavioral Sciences, Tulane University, New Orleans, LA, USA

J. Pien et al. (eds.), *Onward*,
https://doi.org/10.1007/978-3-032-15776-8_2

I can't bear it, to treat a patient without knowing who they are.

I can't stomach the emptiness.

I managed to uncover a remote alcohol history that could explain the "incidental" nodular liver on his CT from admission. I learned that he lived by himself—no, actually, he lived with his cat. I learned that he didn't expect any visitors, and he joked that his grandkids don't care about him when I asked.

I always ask about visitors. I have to know how alone my patients will be, as they sit in a room waiting indefinitely for the next healthcare worker to appear.

The techs were gone for 2 minutes; I'd barely placed my stethoscope on his chest when they returned. He had been too weak and uncomfortable to sit up so I could reach his back. They started moving him to the stretcher, and without thinking, I spent the last few seconds I had doing one thing I always do: I slipped off his socks.

I always take off my patient's socks.

I always take off my patient's socks, and I always ask permission first.

I ask permission to take off my patient's socks, and so far, I've never had someone refuse. Of course I ask permission before doing any exam, but it's usually more a statement than a question—"I'm going to listen to your heart now, okay?"

But not with the socks. With the socks, I truly ask.

"Is it alright if I take your socks off?"

And I don't move. I don't start before they answer. I stand at the foot of their bed, and I don't go near their socks until they say I can. It makes them feel respected and cared for—and it puts me in a lower, humbler role—when I take their socks off.

Once they reply, I carefully roll the tops down and gently lift the heels as I slip each sock beneath. I slow down as I reach the toes, because I've discovered that a lot of people have dry feet, and sometimes the nails will snag, and I don't want to hurt my patient.

It's an easier thing for them to consent to. I've had many patients struggle to sit forward so I can auscultate their lungs, and I've had many patients squirm around in bed to lie flat while I palpate their abdomen.

But I can take off most anyone's socks without being much of a bother.

After I've been granted permission and the socks are off, I check the pulses—and while I check the pulses, I inspect the feet. It distracts the patient when I check the pulses, so they don't become self-conscious about me staring at their feet—they don't realize I'm inspecting. I always check for edema, because so many people have volume overload. And I always check sensation, because so many people have diabetes.

It reminds me, too, to ask about their baseline and their standard care.

"Are your feet normally swollen like this?"

"Oh, you see someone for your neuropathy?"

I look at the toenails. Sometimes an old lady has bright pink nail polish, and I smile and tell her how pretty it is, and she smiles back and, for a moment, we talk about something unrelated to illness. Sometimes there's fungus. Other times, there are bruises or missing nails. Maybe ulcers. Maybe the skin is very thick, maybe cracked and flaking. Maybe the feet are nice and healthy and soft. Maybe there's a tan line at the ankle, and I learn my patient is a gardener or a runner.

So there my patient was, in mid-air, moving from the bed to the stretcher by the technicians' steady hands. I slipped off his socks, and I didn't have time to do everything I normally would, but I did have time to see the bulging pocket of pus, maybe two or three centimeters long, on the dorsum of his right foot.

"Does your right foot hurt?"

The techs slid the door open to wheel him into the hall.

"No."

"This wound on your foot—how long have you had it?"

We were completely out of the room now.

"I don't know, maybe a few weeks. It doesn't hurt."

They were rushing him away from me.

"Do you know how you got it?" I was hurrying after them.

"I think my cat scratched me. Or maybe it got hurt putting on my shoes, because my feet have been so big—"

He was right, they were quite edematous.

"—but I'm not sure."

And he was gone. He was gone before I could ask more, see more, listen and touch and investigate more. He was gone before the intern could see him and before the senior resident could see him. It was just me, and I doubted myself as I gave my report.

"He had a purulent wound on his right foot."

"Purulent? Are you sure it wasn't just dead skin?" The senior resident was trying to be helpful.

My heart began pounding. I wasn't sure. I wasn't sure at all. It had happened so fast—I could very easily be misremembering it. Wow, my heart was pounding. No, I wasn't sure.

"I'm pretty sure. I mean, there was pus, so that's purulent, right? I'm sorry, it was so quick. They were putting him on the bed to go to imaging when I showed up. I only had a few minutes. I think it was purulent, but I didn't have a good chance to really look or talk to him or anything. He said it might've been his cat."

The attending also had her doubts. When we went to his room, he was still gone. He was somewhere else in the maze of the hospital, wherever the techs had delivered him, while we stood there in the hall trying to decide if the anxious medical student with the high-pitched voice and the bright orange ribbon in her hair had any idea what she was talking about.

So we left and went to see our other patients in that building. Two hours later, we were walking away, headed to North Tower to see the rest of the list, when I heard myself speak up.

"What about the new patient who was at ultrasound?" I immediately regretted it. They were going to see how clueless I was, that I didn't even know what "purulent" looks like.

"Right!" The attending stopped. "Let's go see if he's back." My heart started pounding again. At least I'd already done the presentation—we just needed to lay eyes on him.

We walked in. The attending introduced herself and wasted no time before looking at his right foot. She turned to me, and I braced for the verbal lashing.

"Go get his nurse, and grab a wound culture kit from the supply closet."

I was frozen for a second. "Is that purulent?" I was confused. Hadn't I been wrong?

"Yeah," she half-laughed, "that's purulent."

Later, once the culture was sent and we again walked towards the North Tower, she looked at me: "That's a hell of a hallway exam you did."

Wait. Was that…a compliment? Praise? Did I do something *right*?

"I—I always take the socks off," I stuttered. I shrugged.

That afternoon, my senior resident and intern bragged about it in the resident workroom. They had identified the admitting resident from the night before—the one who had admitted our patient without noticing the blatantly infected wound on the top of his right foot.

"Our medical student found it!" They teased.

"You missed it, and the *medical student* found it!"

"She took his socks off!"

Everyone laughed and looked at me.

"I, you know—I always take the socks off." I shrugged again.

It became his principal problem. The culture grew *Serratia marcescens*, and the antibiotics worked beautifully. But the Lasix didn't work beautifully. And the Bumex didn't work beautifully.

It was complicated; I began stumbling over the differential each morning. He had cirrhosis, probably from that alcohol history I'd discovered. He also had raging rheumatoid arthritis, and his Remicade didn't put him in the best position when we started talking about infection. There was a pericardial effusion, too, which of course could be from anything—but it might not have been enough for a pericardiocentesis, and we didn't know if it'd be worth draining anyway, since it could easily come back depending on what was causing it in the first place. And we were pretty sure the acute kidney injury was prerenal, until his creatinine jumped to four-point-something on Hospital Day 4, and I reminded my senior resident he'd gotten contrast 4 days ago.

"I've been keeping track of it in the note," I said. "Just in case. See?" And I showed her the problem list, where I kept copy-pasting a set of parentheses that read: (Of note, pt received Omnipaque on admission).

Nothing was straightforward. Infectious Disease didn't know, Rheumatology didn't know, Nephrology didn't know, Cardiology didn't know.

We didn't know.

But my patient—he knew. Not what was happening, but how it was going to end, even before we did.

"Apparently my grandkids care about me," he joked, but there was a real love in his voice. I knew they cared about him—we updated his granddaughter every day.

On Hospital Day 2, I learned his cat was named Bella. We talked about Bella often. I teared up with him the day before he started dialysis when he told me that she was going to go live with his six-year-old great-granddaughter.

"She can take better care of Bella," he said.

Nephrology had declared him to be a poor candidate for dialysis. They were right. We'd already talked about code status, and he'd put together a will. On Hospital Day 9, all he wanted was Bella. "I miss my dog," I shared. "We sure love animals, don't we?"

He agreed, and I didn't even ask how he was doing. We both knew it was a pointless question, so we talked about Bella. On Hospital Day 10, he died.

They let his family bring Bella to see him right before—he was wrong that first day, when he told me he wouldn't have any visitors.

He always said "Merry Christmas!" when I (or anyone) left his room. He only ever snapped at me once, and I didn't mind; he was in pain. He let me take his socks off every time I asked. He told me—proudly, frequently—how much he spoiled Bella. He remembered me, amidst all the nurses and techs and consults, and I remembered him—every morning, I opened his chart first.

And I'll remember him.

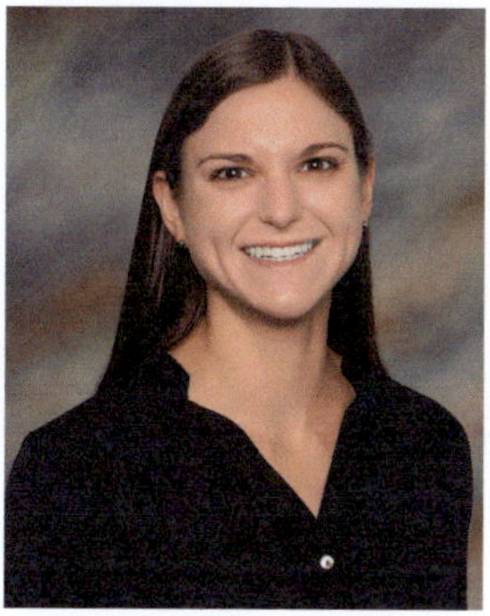

Alexandra Belardo-DeFelice earned her MD from the University of Virginia School of Medicine and is currently a psychiatry resident at Tulane University in her home state of Louisiana. She has special interest in trauma- and stressor-related disorders, clinical ethics, and reproductive psychiatry. As a military spouse, she especially enjoys working with the military population. She writes both prose and poetry, and her work has been featured in narrative medicine journals such as *Intima*, *Pulse*, and *Hektoen International*.

Blue Tennis Shoes

3

Megan Campany

There is nothing quite like the quiet efficiency of a hospital early in the morning. Long before the rest of the world and the patients are awake, our team is already at work. It's a subtle kind of hustle, a rhythm born from repetition. Vitals, I&Os, labs, and overnight events. We "run" the list—it's just that… a tempo that maintained to accomplish an insurmountable workload in an incredibly short period of time. The efficiency is a necessity and a practice—it functions undisturbed, punctuated with quick sips of coffee, the quiet clicks of a mouse, and the scratch of a pen. Occasionally, an irregularity in the form of an abnormal result pulls us forward towards the screen, sitting a little straighter, a little more awake. Not critical, something to check on later that day… and back into the routine we go.

I was no exception to the tempo that day. A little bleary-eyed, I folded my patient list, tucked it in my back pocket, and headed out of the workroom to lay eyes on my patients. I leaned against the back wall in the elevator, stifled a yawn, and pulled out the already

First presented for the Kalanthi Writing Award, 2023

M. Campany (✉)
Division of Cardiothoracic Surgery, Department of Surgery, University of North Carolina at Chapel Hill, Chapel Hill, NC, USA
e-mail: megan.campany@unchealth.unc.edu

J. Pien et al. (eds.), *Onward*,
https://doi.org/10.1007/978-3-032-15776-8_3

wrinkled list, scanning for the details of my first patient to check on. I hadn't seen her yet—my co-resident had been managing her care over the last few days. According to the notes, she was a 26-year-old female with a long-standing history of Crohn's disease that came into the hospital two days before with a bowel obstruction. Tucked into the bottom line of the text box, someone had typed "f/u CT with scope" … medical jargon for bad news. She had undergone the scope yesterday and confirmed what we already knew to be true—there was a tumor that had grown enough to partially block her intestines and create the obstruction causing her pain. It wasn't all that surprising—years of constant inflammation is the perfect nidus for a cancer to begin to grow. *Such a shame*, I remember thinking. *She's so young*.

It wasn't my place to tell her the details yet—we would wait for more senior members of our team to review the images and pathology reports before developing a treatment plan. It would include a large surgery, likely chemo or immunotherapy. Her whole life was about to change… but *would I still be on service when they did her operation? Maybe this time I could oversew the anastomosis?*

My thoughts were far from her blithe situation as I gently tapped on the door and pushed it open. We see patients with illnesses far more critical than hers every single day—truthfully, I wasn't affected by it. I simply needed to ask the same two questions everyone else on my patient list would hear from me this morning… "how's your pain?" followed by the fan-favorite, "have you passed gas yet?" I flipped on the lights—there's no subtle way to wake someone before 5 AM—and ran through the usual interaction, fully on autopilot. Her pain was well controlled… maybe a 2/10. She'd had a few watery bowel movements following the procedure yesterday. I scribbled this down, gave her belly a cursory press, and turned for the door, ready to step across the hall to my next patient. Out of the corner of my eye, I noticed a pair of blue tennis shoes tucked neatly in the corner, perfectly aligned with each other. The same ones, in fact, that I had on my own feet. I'd found them on sale a few weeks back and made the impulse purchase, only to find that they pinched my smallest toe when I walked too fast.

I wonder if they pinch her toe, too?

That was all it took. A pair of tennis shoes, and I was jolted from the routine I found so much comfort in. That rhythm of efficiency and hustle and repetition was shattered.

Because not only did this young woman have my tennis shoes… she had my disease too.

I had been diagnosed with Crohn's disease early in medical school. The first few times I saw patients with a complication from their—our—disease, I had felt a little jolt in my stomach. But those patients were older, probably didn't keep as good control over their disease, hadn't had the access to immediate care like I had. At least that's what I told myself to keep moving, to keep pace, to keep distance. Eventually, I numbed to it, and now I hardly even notice. But that morning, on 7-East in the room furthest down on the right, I found myself staring right into the eyes of my disease. It looked like a brunette, a few weeks past her 26th birthday with "concerning findings" on a scan. It looked like a massive surgery, cycles of chemotherapy, months of recovery.

It looked like a pair of blue tennis shoes… and it terrified me. What was it that separated her from me? How did she end up in that bed, on my to-do list, in the middle of my morning routine?

How could I make sure that I didn't?

…

Being both a provider and a patient is an interesting dynamic. You see both sides—the medical knowledge provides a deeper understanding of the disease itself, the pathophysiology, the mechanism behind the drugs that mitigate the symptoms, and the complications that seem to always arise. You see the statistics and the exceptions, and occasionally you glimpse the human that exists in between.

But as the patient—you know the weeks and months of waiting for appointments. You see the days between those appointments with symptoms that never quite seem to relent, that permeate into every aspect of normal life. You live the hours on hold with insurance companies, the labs and tests and bills. You become the person attempting to live with the disease, desperately and quietly asking to learn to thrive with it.

I had always thought this was to my advantage. Being both a provider and a patient allowed an empathy with my patients that not everyone could understand. I knew that Sara in Building 2 could draw labs so quickly you didn't even notice the stick. I knew that the pharmacy was open until 6, but if Ben was working, you could pick up medications at 6:15. I knew that the second aisle in Target carried the best candy to make a bowel prep easier, and that the Japanese place on Seventh Street had the best broth for a clear liquid diet. My tips and tricks had become secrets of my trade… and somehow that made it worth it. Sure, being a patient was frustrating and overwhelming and challenging, but it also made me a better doctor… so it had to be worth it.

Except for today.

Today, it threatened to break me. Sure, I knew Sara in the lab and Ben in the pharmacy and where to get the best soup, but I also knew what her next six months would look like. I knew how brutal the surgery would be, how much it would hurt, how much her life was about to change. The problem, I realized, as I looked down at the pair of shoes forgotten by the door, had nothing to do with what I knew.

It was what I didn't know.

I didn't know how to avoid becoming her.

I glanced back over my shoulder to find that she was already fast asleep again. As I had been so well trained to do, I tucked the emotion down, quieted it, and walked out the door, closing it quietly behind me. I leaned against the wall, no longer bleary-eyed and tired. Reality had come on a little too quickly for my liking that morning.

I took a deep breath and pulled out the same crinkled list. Next patient… a 52-year-old woman with a gallbladder that was no longer satisfied with its place in her abdomen. I crossed the hall, knocked on the door, and turned on the light.

I wish I could tell you that I had some big revelation that day. That she changed my practice, or the way I treat my patients. In reality, I rotated off service and didn't follow her surgery or recovery after. In truth—I've been too afraid to pull up her chart and check. But I haven't worn those shoes again. They sit on a shelf in my closet, collecting dust as I collect years of training, a daily reminder of all that I have to lose, and occasionally of all that I have to give.

So, I continue to hustle. I have to get lost in the efficiency, the routine, the training. It's the only way to survive, to breathe, to keep going in a marathon like this. But every now and then, I see a pair of blue tennis shoes, and I pause.

When I least expect it, I see it.

The human behind the diagnosis code. The wife and daughter and sister and friend. The person.

And I think it's moments like this that remind me of the human I'm supposed to be becoming as I work for the MD behind my name, the title of surgeon on my jacket. In a field that demands you keep pace, I remember to pause. I remember a pair of blue tennis shoes. And then I go see the next patient.

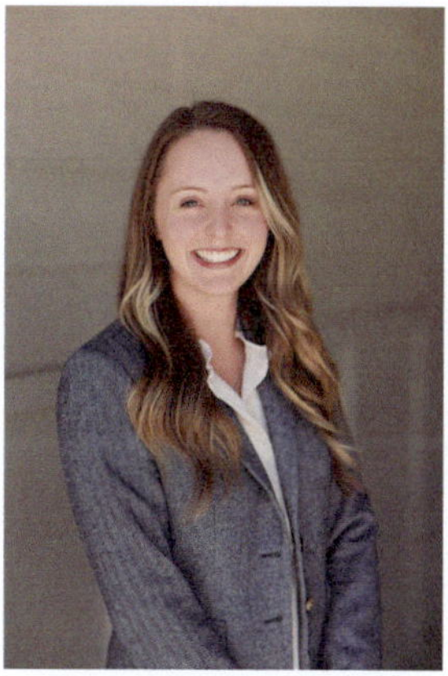

Megan Campany MD, MS, is a current resident in Cardiothoracic Surgery at the University of North Carolina at Chapel Hill. She plans to focus her future practice on minimally invasive thoracic oncology as well as lung transplantation. Her medical career first began in the mountains of North Carolina while pursuing a degree in Exercise Physiology and working in an autonomic performance laboratory focusing on children with Down Syndrome. She proceeded to complete medical school at the Mayo Clinic Alix School of Medicine in Scottsdale, Arizona, while concurrently receiving a master's degree in Health Care Policy and Administration from Arizona State University. She remains an active researcher with focuses in esophageal and lung cancer, lung transplantation, and oncologic disparities. In her spare time, she enjoys trying new restaurants with her family and friends, cooking, taking her dog to explore new places, and exercising.

4 On ECMO and Ubers

Hannah Decker

It had been a long week. Our attending smiled wanly as we made evening rounds in the intensive care nursery, saying to nobody in particular, "If we are going to put this baby on ECMO, it would be ideal if it wasn't in between the hours of midnight and 4 AM."

It only took me a few years of residency to learn that hoping to sleep through the night is dangerous—the more strongly you yearn for uninterrupted sleep, the nearer the certainty that it won't happen. So, I was unsurprised when my phone buzzed me awake that night with a text message. "We are going to proceed with ECMO shortly if you want to come." I splashed some water on my face and changed out of my pajamas. Despite knowing how dangerous it is to drive while tired, the convenience of taking my own car to the hospital was hard to shake. But it was the first rotation of a new academic year and I had promised my husband I would be more cautious. I called an Uber, watching instructional videos of ECMO cannulation, while I waited for it to arrive. Already dreading rounds the next morning, I tried my best to get a few more minutes of rest en route, but I was unsettled thinking of the baby and his family.

First published in Intima: A Journal of Narrative Medicine.

H. Decker (✉)
Department of Surgery, University of California San Francisco,
San Francisco, CA, USA
e-mail: hannah.decker@ucsf.edu

J. Pien et al. (eds.), *Onward*,
https://doi.org/10.1007/978-3-032-15776-8_4

To be honest, I was unsettled by much of my pediatric surgery rotation. If I truly stopped to think about the situation of many of these families who lived in the hospital, caregiving for seriously ill children, it brought me to my knees. During the days, I tried to avoid this line of thinking, hustling to take care of our large census of children. But at night, my patients' names and faces swam through my mind. A teenager with a nasogastric tube in for weeks, calmly doing homework in the hospital armchair. A mother, eyes welling up: "Do you really have to do the surgery tomorrow? It is my birthday and I just don't want anything bad to happen." A young girl in the pediatric intensive care unit, swollen with steroids, whose skin shredded like wet tissues when we placed a central line. A baby who swallowed something not meant to be swallowed. Her grandmother's face when we told her it meant an emergent operation. A precocious teenager with metastatic disease who wanted to become a doctor like me. A usually stoic 14-year-old, immunosuppressed from treatment for cancer, crying big, salty tears after we completed a bedside incision and drainage—from the pain, or perhaps from the unfairness of it all. I have a 14-year-old brother. He is usually stoic, too.

When I arrived that night, the neonatal intensive care unit was swarming with activity. Each team member was diligently doing their job, in the middle of the night, to give this little one a shot at what can only be described as a very challenging first day in this world.

Our team proceeded with cannulation under the heat lamps of the NICU. Even with loupes on, the beating anatomy seemed impossibly small. Finally, the circuit was connected. The team began to breathe a little easier and, eventually, dissipate. Weary, I called an Uber home. As the car started, I began to doze off. A few minutes into the ride, I was awoken by a question. "Do you work in the children's hospital?"

I explained that I was a surgical resident working there for the month.

"Do you know any of the pediatric perfusion nurses?"

I was startled by the question, having had just spent all night closely working with them. "Yes, I know some of them. Why?"

He looked at me in the rearview mirror, and the words tumbled out as we drove through the sleeping streets. As it turns out, a long time ago, his infant son had been on ECMO for many days. The perfusion nurses were a constant accompaniment at the bedside. He had gotten to know them as they carefully watched and troubleshot the machine keeping his son alive—and in turn, they had grown to love his son. He smiled as he told me how they had burned a CD of music that the family loved and played it for his son so that he could feel at home, even when his parents couldn't be there.

The man grew quiet, as if deciding to tell me more. "My son died fourteen years ago this month. Every year, for fourteen years, something happens during this season that makes me think of him – remember him. This year, it is you, getting in my car."

He thanked me for learning how to take care of sick children. I thanked him for sharing the story of his son with me. Soon, the ride was over. I slowly made my way up my stairs and into my bed.

The next morning back in the NICU, I relayed his words to the perfusion nurses. They remembered him. They had loved, and subsequently mourned, his son all those years ago. His name and face swam in their head, too. They told me their stories over the soft whirring of this ECMO circuit, for this baby, loved by these parents.

These kinds of moments are the ones we carry. The ones when the universe reminds us—even though it is a struggle, and we are exhausted, and our patients break our hearts—why we do what we do. For the life in front of us now. For the faces and names that swim in our heads. For the families of those faces and names who remember.

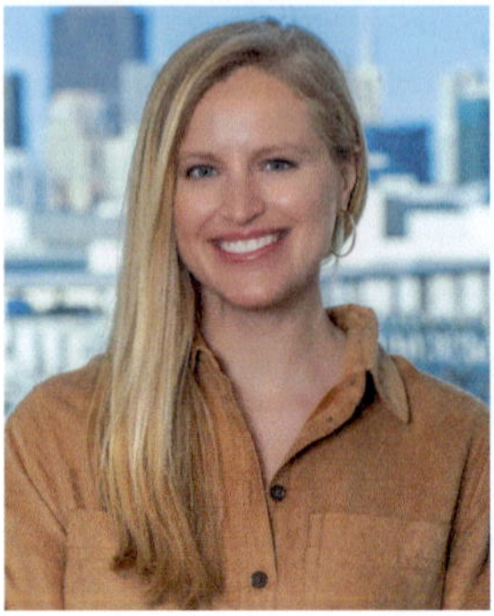

Hannah Decker is a general surgery resident at UCSF and health services researcher interested in improving access to high-quality surgical care for vulnerable populations. Before getting her medical degree at Emory University School of Medicine, she studied history at Dartmouth College. Writing fiction and creative non-fiction has been an essential part of her medical training, allowing her to process the moving and challenging experiences that accompany learning to be a doctor.

Cold Coffee and Histology Slides

5

Rebecca Grossman-Kahn

Welcome to the Cancer Center. There is a small hallway that juts off the main thoroughfare—just before you reach the café—in the hospital where I was a medical student. I sped through this hallway hundreds of times, bouncing between lecture halls and the cafeteria, between small group learning and afternoons shadowing in a clinic. There is a sign at the turn-off, above the doorframe that says, "Welcome to the Cancer Center." I walked by this sign every day for 2 years and never really noticed it.

"Welcome to the Cancer Center," announces a semi-professional actor to a large group of second-year medical students gathered in a conference room. This is the name of the short play we are about to observe. We have 2 hours reserved in our curriculum to learn how to break bad news to patients. The actors perform a piece following a woman through her diagnosis with colon cancer. The teaching points are painfully obvious: medical jargon flows more smoothly than a comforting phrase from the resident's lips; the providers don't see the patient's harried exchange with the front desk about insurance coverage; the patient's face lights up when the warm, wise attending finally asks the patient about what brings her joy.

R. Grossman-Kahn (✉)
Psychiatry, HealthPartners, St Paul, MN, USA

J. Pien et al. (eds.), *Onward*,
https://doi.org/10.1007/978-3-032-15776-8_5

Next, it is our turn. We break into small groups so each student can practice telling an actor bad news. This shouldn't be too hard, we think, scanning the prompts printed out. We are all wearing our short white coats as we were instructed, a costume for the part.

In one scene, my 22-year-old classmate wearing a sagging white coat has to tell the actor, Steve, that his wife died in a car accident. Steve pounds the walls of the room and collapses to the floor while tears stream down all of our faces. My classmate timidly gets on the ground next to Steve, barely in arm's reach. He tentatively reaches for Steve's shoulder to give it a pat, scanning the audience's eyes for help, for clues. His partner, another classmate, shuts down and freezes, unable to say anything at all.

It is my turn. I pull the chair closer to Steve in order to calmly tell him that his daughter has just been diagnosed with diabetes. As I begin to talk, he looks down and intently cleans his glasses on the hem of his shirt. The actors are trained to goad us, to lead us to the limits of our patience and compassion. Before I know it, Steve is asking whether I'll be informing his ex-wife of the diagnosis and begins to list her many character flaws. I let a smile slip. But only because I know this is pretend, can't he see? We leave the conference room shaken, doubting our ability to ever provide comfort, much less expertise. I replay my scene over in my head as I blankly stare at histology slides later that day. Surely we'll do better with real patients.

A few months later, on morning rounds at the hospital, my team is seeing an elderly patient who came in to the hospital because he fell; imaging we did showed a terminal cancer. It is my classmate's job to relay these imaging results to the patient. The teaching team files into his room, ducking beneath the thin curtain separating him from his roommate.

"Sir, remember those pictures we took of your liver?" My classmate's voice quivers. "Um, we found something" (pause). "That we are very worried about."

How do you teach a student to say the words that will shatter someone's life?

"Give it to me straight." He is sitting on the side of the bed, turning his good ear towards my classmate's faint voice.

"We found a mass…"

"—cancer," the attending physician interrupts. "We found *cancer*."

No wonder we call it breaking bad news. It is snapping a stick in half, shattered pieces that can never be one piece again.

We never spoke about how patients have to break the bad news, too. This is the lesson I learn when I flew home between exams a few months later. My mother took me on a walk to get coffee, and as we were leaving the house said, "I have news. My mammogram was suspicious. I've had more tests. I have to go to the oncologist." What I remember is liquid heat spread slowly through my body. We eventually made it to the coffee shop. I could not drink anything, emotion constricting my throat, and brought the cold coffee back home, setting it on the counter.

I had just learned about breast cancer as part of our second-year curriculum. I dutifully studied the purple-patterned calcifications on a pathology slide. I answered multiple-choice questions. One in eight women by the time they turn 80. I had memorized a pathway for treatment, but I didn't have any comforting answers to my mother's questions. I was horrified. I had studied it all with such nonchalance.

I accompanied my mother to her first appointment in a slick new building. She wore a new gray suit and orange scarf. In her early 60s, she had just recently begun wearing high heels to match her new job. I kept thinking she belongs in her office right now, not here. We acted out the motions of getting into the elevator and pushing the button to the Oncology floor. A sign pointing the way: *Welcome to the Cancer Center*. I glared back at it, annoyed at its gall to welcome us there, as if we had a choice. My mother became the one in eight women who swipes her credit card on a co-pay to see an oncologist, and it feels like it isn't real.

"It will just be a blip in your year; really, an excellent prognosis," insisted her new doctor. "After all, it is *proliferation of malignant epithelial cells completely contained within breast ducts not thought to be metastatic*." My mother looked to me. I recognized the words, but what did they mean? A *blip*? How could I have spent 2 years learning so much about medicine and know so little?

I realized that until then, I had been learning medicine as if it were a foreign language. The first 2 years of med school taught me how to sound out vocabulary words—*clonal population of atypical cohesive cells confined to ducts and lobules*. I rolled the foreign phrases around in my mouth like hard candies. I memorized flashcards, even silly mnemonics, all just symptoms floating out of context. I had learned to read the medicine book out loud, but I couldn't explain the plot.

Where was the missing Learning Objective in that breast cancer lecture?

- *At the end of this lecture, students will understand:*
  The patient will spend months in agony knowing she can't stop her body from feeding the malignant cells.

Where were the slides about the patient's matted hair after surgery? We were never quizzed on what it feels like to hear "eight centimeters" when in your head the cancer was a tiny bead the size of this *o*.

How do you teach a student the weight of their new vocabulary words?

No matter how many years we spend studying textbooks, nothing can prepare us for the hospital. Clinical years become the study abroad program to practice our new language, our cultural immersion into the messy hospital workrooms, where we gain conversational proficiency. For 2 years, I was shielded from this side of medicine while I learned lists of diagnoses, detached from their meaning to the humans who receive them.

I wish I had a pocket dictionary to translate between textbook information, what attendings say behind closed doors, and what patients experience after we leave the room. I imagine how I might have annotated my medical school books for my past self. Pulmonary embolism: *Your attending will spend days obsessing over oxygen saturations. Your patient will eventually tearfully tell you he thought he was going to die when he couldn't breathe on the way to the hospital.*

Thyroidectomy: *post-surgery, the first time a mother will ever smell sour to her daughter.* Prostate abscess: *an estranged son will bring his delirious, septic Dad into the ICU and wonder if he'll lose him before they can repair their relationship.* Fibromuscular dysplasia: *Your team will struggle to find the cause of the strokes. Your patient's husband will bring his wife daily lattés, desperate to see her smile, and spoon her the sweet foam after she loses her ability to sip from a cup.* Ductal carcinoma in situ: the oncologist will call it "just a blip in the life," but your mother will still want you by her side, even with your floating, fragmented M3 knowledge.

At the end of this lecture, students will understand: behind every diagnostic histology slide we breeze through in the next hour, there is a restless grandfather twisting his sheets; a woman sitting in her car in the parking garage, crying too hard to drive home; a family wandering the hospital halls late at night, looking for a coffee that will go cold, undrunk.

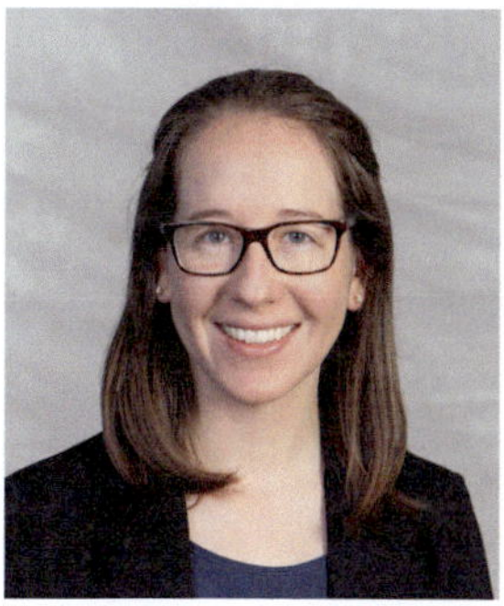

Rebecca Grossman-Kahn is a writer and physician based in Minneapolis, where she practices emergency psychiatry. Her work has been published in *The New England Journal of Medicine*, *Bellevue Literary Review*, the *Intima*, and *The Examined Life Journal*. She is a graduate of Stanford University and University of Michigan Medical School.

The Manic Patient: "Refusing Labs"

6

Rachel H. Han

I was looking forward to having Memorial Day weekend off. It was Friday, and we—the medical students rotating on general surgery—had just been informed that we were expected to round on our postoperative patients on at least one day over the long weekend. I suppose I should have always expected to work the weekend, especially since I scrubbed in on the partial colectomy that morning, but alas, my delusional optimism had kicked in again. I bargained with the other third-year medical student, Alex, to work Saturday so that I wouldn't have to miss another Sunday church service.

I have missed so many Sundays because of medical school, so I'm quick to recognize an opportunity to seize a hospital-free Sunday when I get one. To me, Sunday is more than just a day off; it's the one day I find peace and comfort. As a Korean American, I was late to appreciate the fellowship offered to me at Asian-American churches. Before medical school, I'd never realized how much having a community that looks like me could remind me of home, and how much they—a community of familiar-appearing strangers—could anchor me securely to my treasured

First published in the Pegasus Review

R. H. Han (✉)
Psychiatry, Walter Reed National Military Medical Center,
Bethesda, MD, USA

J. Pien et al. (eds.), *Onward*,
https://doi.org/10.1007/978-3-032-15776-8_6

identity and lifelong values. Now that most of my week is spent at the hospital surrounded by people who do not look like me, Sundays with my church community feel all the more sacred.

Alex is kind; he is happy to work on Sunday. I figure it is not so bad anyways, since on Saturday I could also carpool to work with my friend, Jon, another medical student who was already planning to work as well—it's amazing how small my victories have become. I ask Jon for a ride, and he responds that he plans to leave for work at 4:15 a.m.—a whole hour earlier than I needed to be in by. I am not what they call a 'morning person.' *Big sigh.* But this is all fine. I signed up for this. Whatever.

Saturday morning arrives, and I am looking up my patient's vital signs and preparing to pre-round. My phone buzzes. I place my phone face down. The buzzing continues—it's a call. *Jon? What does he want now? He's so impatient.*

"What's up?" I whisper. I don't know why I whispered; it's 5:00 a.m., and I'm alone in the surgery clinic. It's still dark out. I could burp, and no one would hear it. (I was nauseated from acid reflux throughout my surgery rotation.)

"Can you come talk to my patient? She only speaks Korean and the residents gave up on her."

Gave up? How?

"Shouldn't you call an official interpreter?"

"They said they already tried."

"Mhm… Sure they did."

"Well, they've moved on from her and are too busy to care… Just come… please."

"Okay, fine."

I feel guilty for my reluctance, but then again I had not completed looking up my own patient's morning labs, let alone seen my patient yet. I needed to be prepared for rounds by 6:00 a.m., and I know the chief resident will use this presentation to evaluate me for the rotation. He has not been the type to 'pimp' in the OR, which has, unfortunately, led me to wonder whether staying up the extra hours to prep for cases is even worth it. Yes, I do acknowledge that the extra work is probably good for my education (lifelong learning *blah*), but perhaps it's also contributing to my increased irritability and lack of interest in communicating with family. These sentiments are especially strong when I catch up with classmates who brag about how little they study and how well they perform. Jon always reminds me that "comparison is the thief of joy," yet I can't help how I feel.

I show up on the medicine floor, and Jon waves me over. He fills me in; the patient was admitted for toxic overdose of an unknown substance, has a history of bipolar disorder, and is refusing labs. I think to myself, "Do I know any Korean person with bipolar disorder?"

I enter the room and greet the patient in Korean with an awkward head bob to *insah*. I have her attention. She turns to my friend and says, "You again!" Then, as if I am someone she has known for ages, she directs her energy to me and proceeds to tell me about how my tall white friend has been bothering her all morning and how she does not trust all the young kids running this place. Jon stands there blankly, oblivious to her commentary and waiting expectantly. She motions for me to draw nearer. "Don't tell anyone but I have special powers." She smirks as she confides in me that she can look directly at the sun. She reaches for my hand. "Do you like *kimchi?* I can make *kimchi!*" I learn that her daughter is a fan; however, her husband, a Japanese American, does not appreciate the smell.

"Do they know you're here?" I ask.

My question goes unanswered. I notice that she is suddenly tearful. I remember learning about emotional lability, and yet I don't know how to respond to the reality of the definition unraveling before me. Uncomfortable with silence, I slide in a few sentences on how important it is for us to check her labs, which requires drawing her blood—the real reason I was called here to speak with her.

"I am weak and have very little blood to give," she responds.

The way she speaks of her health is familiar—I see my mother in her, worrying about my cold hands and poor circulation. I emphasize again how important the blood draw is for her survival. She nods in acceptance. I signal to my friend, who immediately excuses himself to fetch a tech.

While the tech fumbles around preparing to draw her blood, the patient has her eyes glued on me. She asks me who I am. Only now do I notice that she has both of her hands wrapped around mine. Before answering, I hesitate, recalling what I had been taught about sharing too much about our personal lives with patients, *especially psych patients*. But I guess this is my first lesson on countertransference, because I cannot resist the urge to give her something that would allow her to perhaps bask in reflected glory. I tell her that I am a medical student and was born in the States. My parents first immigrated to California before settling in New Jersey, across the bridge from New York City. I have an older brother. My mom is in her fifties and just started to make her own *kimchi* at home. She used to buy it from the church, where the eldresses prepared and sold *kimchi* to raise funds for the women's ministry. But the eldresses have started to feel their age, and the next generations of women do not want to make *kimchi*—it's hard work to make in bulk. Now, they raise funds by selling homemade nut clusters and other *banchan*.

The patient is surprised when she notices the tech packing up.

"*Han guh yah*?"

"*Neh*, he's already done!" I reply.

It's 5:50 a.m. I have 10 minutes until rounds. I *insah* goodbye and wish her good health. I bolt out to use a computer at the nurses' station to finish looking up a few more lab values for my post-op patient. I can tell the nurses are suspicious of me. I flip my ID badge to be more visible. I try to be quick. Just need to check one… more… thing… Got it. Five minutes until rounds. I run upstairs. Quick small talk with the post-op patient. Overnight events? Pain? Did you walk? Heart and lungs within normal limits. Wound check. Done. Foldable clipboard in hand, I present the status of my post-op patient to the chief resident.

He interrupts my every other sentence. His feedback is vague, boorish, and typical, stuff like "speak up and be more confident!" At this point, a small piece of the hidden curriculum of medical school is clear to me: it would be a better use of my time to work on correcting *how* I say something versus *what* I say. I (hate myself for this but) thank him for the feedback! And follow him into the patient's room so that he can validate what I presented and inform the patient that, unfortunately, he can't go home today.

I am released after rounds and speed walk to the locker room to change out of my scrubs before anyone is able to invite me to stay and watch an "interesting case" (in the corner, out of the way, that is). I am in the clear. I look outside, and the sun is up. My weekend starts now!

On my way out of the hospital, I call a rideshare. I have 5 minutes to kill. It has been over a week since I called home, and I finally have a story to share. I usually call my mom; it's reflexive. I don't know why, but this time, I decide to call my dad.

He picks up on the first ring. I tell him about my morning events. He laughs at how early I had to wake up, reminiscing about the days when he would have to wake me up on Saturday mornings by blasting Janet Jackson from the living room downstairs. When I start to tell him about the Korean patient, he goes quiet. I expect him to respond with pride about raising a Korean-speaking daughter in America. Instead, I hear him sigh.

"How can she think to kill herself?"

Though I should have known better as a Korean American, I realize that I had just stepped into a big pile of steaming Korean taboo. I forgot that suicide and mental health, in general, are not commonly talked about outside of the hospital. These topics are avoided even more in Korean communities, not excluding my family. Immediately sensing his discomfort, I—now also uncomfortable—say something thoughtless about how often I have interacted with suicidal patients in medical school. It doesn't comfort him. I then blab on about how special I felt for being able to use my mother tongue. Still, I can tell the damage is done; my story upset him. I ruined his day, and he is going to dwell on death, lost family members, and aging. I can picture him entering our home through the garage door tonight, a little after 8:00 p.m., going upstairs to wash his face, coming downstairs, and immediately walking over to the dining room for a drink to pair with dinner.

I can't stop thinking about the fact that I won't be home to undo the damage and distract him from this downward spiral and remind him of his success through me and my triumphs. I don't want to perpetuate Asian stereotypes, but this is the reality of our home. I have no defense, just anxiety. I use my arriving rideshare as an excuse to hang up, even though I had been in the car for half of this conversation already. I then ruminate over how I should have stuck to our usual short conversations about how well I am doing and how well I am eating (but not too much, I promise).

Growing up, I was often told, "don't tell anyone." My first memory hearing this phrase is as an 8-year-old when my dad was embarrassed that we were staying in a bed and breakfast outside of Paris rather than in a luxury hotel in the city center. I remember also hearing it in high school when my mom forgot I was in the car and worried out loud about how they were going to pay for another semester of college for my brother. And this warning would come after fights that my brother and I had witnessed between our parents. These are the ways that I understood how secrets could exist within our family.

However, it is the secrets that are not said out loud—even at home—that confuse me. While these secrets hang over our heads at the dinner table, my parents give stern nonverbal cues to keep our eyes down. These secrets are hushed when brought up in private. They are the ones I am reminded of months and years later to not share. "You should not even know about this," my mom would say; even though, I obviously already know. I am reminded that if I were to share such secrets about my own family, it would be like lying down supine and spitting because the spit would land on my own face, as a certain Korean proverb says.

In that moment after calling my dad, I did not know how to respond after triggering him. Since then, I have thought much about how I could have responded fully without acknowledging the secret that I knew triggered him. Sometimes I wonder if that's even possible. Further, I wonder if these kinds of secrets will be roadblocks in my endeavors to work with patients from similar cultural backgrounds. These thoughts bring me back to an encounter during my psychiatry rotation with a Hmong patient who was admitted for suicidality, stayed inpatient for over a week, and then was discharged by our team without a clear picture of what his upbringing was like. In our meetings, we gossiped about his silence and were suspicious of his curt responses when answering our questions about his family history. Now, I regret not doing more to create a safe space for him to talk about his home life. I regret not having had the insight to see the potential for progress.

I have recently been made aware that secrets stem from anger, guilt, and shame. In the future, I want to be more direct in pointing out and defining these emotions that my patients may describe or exhibit in order to provide a framework for understanding the triggers of these emotions, perhaps leading us to the secrets. Then, the real work can begin—normalizing emotions and experiences, and relieving the burden of staying silent.

Though over a year has passed, I often think of the manic Korean patient because she is the protagonist of the story that led me to choose psychiatry as my desired medical specialty, and her story has sparked so many conversations with friends and colleagues, my family, and my therapist. I ultimately discovered that her lab results had shown that her liver enzymes were in the thousands. Apparently, she had overdosed on Tylenol—a whole bottle. My mind races when I think of this. *What if I had not been around? What if no one had thought to contact me? What actually happens to patients who 'refuse labs'? Are they pinned down? Sedated? Or blamed for their clinical outcome? What if that clinical outcome is death?* From the conversations that have stemmed from this experience, what is most unsettling to me is how powerless medical students feel because of the way they are observed and evaluated, despite having so much power to make a difference in clinical care given their direct access to patients. Because of how things turned out with her clinical course, I am more confident in asking patients if they are more comfortable speaking in another language and pointing out when an interpreter is needed.

This encounter helped me identify the patient population that I have been missing. Her memory empowered me to initiate a research project to look into the usage of behavioral health resources amongst Asian Americans and Pacific Islanders. Discussing her story provided an opportunity for my Korean-American friend to confide in me about dealing with her mother's suicide attempt that occurred when we were in college together. Her story also helped me identify the role of secrets in my family's culture. Finally, her warmth made me feel useful and needed at a time when my thoughts were consumed with anxiety about taking too long to close port-sites and standing in the way of OB/

GYN residents who were trying to meet numbers for deliveries. I suppose on that day, I was for my patient what my church community is for me: a sweet taste of home, kindness, familiarity, and love, which can often feel so far away in the hospital. In return, my patient, more than anyone else, guided me to my professional 'home'—to work that gives me a sense of belonging.

Disclaimer The opinions and assertions expressed herein are those of the author and do not necessarily reflect the official policy or position of the Uniformed Services University or the Department of Defense.

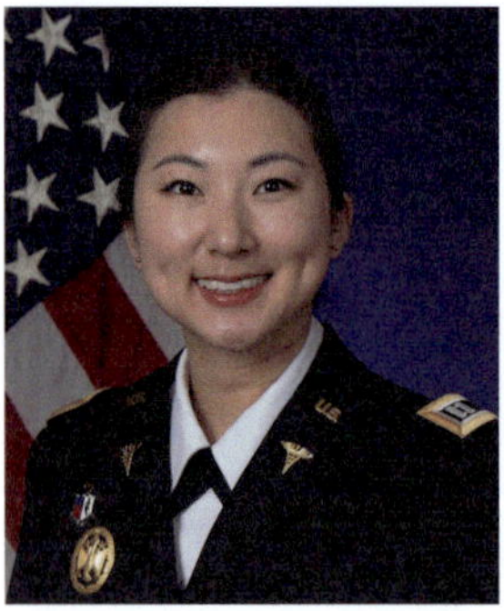

CPT(P) Rachel H. Han MD, is a psychiatrist at Walter Reed National Military Medical Center (WRNMMC) and a Teaching Fellow at the Uniformed Services University of the Health Sciences (USUHS) in Bethesda, Maryland. She earned her Bachelor of Arts degree from Wellesley College and her Doctor of Medicine degree from the F. Edward Hébert School of Medicine at USUHS. She completed her residency in general psychiatry at WRNMMC and her fellowship in addiction psychiatry at New York University. She was the 2020 runner-up for the Irvin D. Yalom Literary Award in prose for her short story, "The Manic Korean Patient: 'Refusing Labs.'"

March Manic

7

Lisa Jacobs

There were 10 pairs of colorful skis standing upright outside my door when I left for my tenth 14-hour overnight shift in 2 weeks.

"I've finally lost it!" I announced to no one. "My psychotic break. It's actually happening."

The nearest slope was half a day away, and I was the only skier in my building. Either the skis magically appeared during my nap or I was hallucinating.

One terrifying lesson of psychiatry is how fast your brain can turn against you. You've been fine your whole life? Doesn't matter. The sanity grounding you to reality can turn to quicksand at any moment. It's like we're all driving around in glass cars. The view's great, but one crash and it can shatter into a million pieces. Reality is frighteningly fragile.

I stood paralyzed like a deer in headlights. Should I report to work if I'm losing my mind? Would the patients notice? My shift was starting in 15 minutes.

I rubbed my eyes. The skis were still there. I reached out to touch one to see if it was real, hand trembling, and they tipped

First published in Intima: A Journal of Narrative Medicine

L. Jacobs (✉)
Department of Psychiatry and Behavioral Sciences, Stanford University School of Medicine, Stanford, CA, USA

J. Pien et al. (eds.), *Onward*,
https://doi.org/10.1007/978-3-032-15776-8_7

over like dominoes, the last few pairs flying down the stairs with a crash.

"These skis are real," I told my neighbor who'd sprinted the stairs to see if I was okay.

"Damn girl, what you been smoking? No shit, they're real," he said. "Sorry to take your hallway. Some guy owed us and this is all he had. Want a pair? You fuck with the snow?"

I'd been trying to save up my measly salary for skis for years, but that's how I got my first pair. Maybe it would be an okay night after all.

Within 30 seconds of entering the psych ER, I knew I was wrong. Three different phone lines were ringing, and 15 patients were on the board, five unseen. Everyone was running around in chaos.

"It's March madness," Chris, the resident signing out to me, said. He looked pale and tired and was devouring a stale turkey sandwich from the patients' fridge, an act of desperation. "It's been like this all day. I'm losing my fucking mind."

He wasn't talking about basketball. March is the worst in psychiatry. One theory is that people who got depressed in the winter finally get the energy to try to kill themselves when the daylight shifts, but it's also prime time for psychosis. Like most things in psychiatry, we know the pattern and how to treat the symptoms, but have no clue why things happen the way they do.

"It's okay," I said. "I thought I had a psychotic break an hour ago."

"I swear I heard voices last night. I actually turned and there was no one there. We're all losing it," Chris said nonchalantly, and then he was gone.

I evaluated 20 patients that night. It was like the *I Love Lucy* episode in the chocolate factory—one gone, two more pile up.

There was a 60-year-old woman with chronic pain who'd just gotten laid off from her secretarial job of 40 years. The police pulled her off a bridge and brought her in against her will. Admitted.

There was a 46-year-old homeless guy, who wrote "suicidal, homicidal, schizophrenic, bipolar" on the intake form, but told me he "really just came to say what's up" because he hadn't been by the ER in a while. Discharged.

There was a 25-year-old guy who was found walking by the train tracks covered in poop, carrying a bunch of rocks, and mumbling. Admitted.

There was a 30-year-old woman who was hearing voices and had been pulled out of the freezing river by police naked, trying to "swim home" to Kansas. Admitted.

The patients were so sick, the staff didn't give me any push-back as I overcrowded our ER with patients awaiting placement.

If you have a stroke or heart attack, you get admitted to the hospital, and we figure out insurance and money later, but if you come in suicidal or psychotic, you sit in the ER, maybe for days, until a hospital reviews your file and agrees to take you. Your insurance must agree to pay first, or the hospital has to agree to charity care. Psych units can reject patients for any reason, most often saying, "nursing is uncomfortable."

By 5 AM, I was beyond any point of exhaustion I had known. I retreated to the call room, a windowless converted office that was 85 degrees with a broken thermostat. A mountain of dirty sheets in the corner stank. There was a rumor of mice. I didn't care. I passed out face down with my shoes on and jumped through the roof when the phone rang like a foghorn 15 minutes later.

"Sorry, doc, got another," the crisis counselor said. I groaned and walked to the office, where he handed me a stack of paperwork and continued, "Easy one. Got out of inpatient today. Has meds, has follow-up, not homeless, not suicidal. Slam-dunk discharge. Just see her quick." She had brought pill bottles containing lithium and antipsychotic tablets for mood stabilization, filled that morning when she got out of the psych unit.

I stumbled out into the loud and rowdy waiting room and saw her dancing in the corner.

"Come with me," I said, and five other patients pointed to themselves hopefully while she kept dancing. I went closer and pointed to her, "You, come with me."

Her name was Aviva, but she told me to call her Abbi or Ilana because "those bitches be the bomb."

"*Broad City*?" I asked, rubbing my eyes. I liked that TV show, too.

Her eyes brightened, and she stood up and started dancing around the interview room. She wasn't at all threatening, so I just let it go. She was humming the show's theme song, saying, "Yaas queen, you're mad Jewey like them and me. Give those ladies a shout! That's what I'm talking about! Abbi's from the Main Line like me. We both do comedy."

"You do comedy?" I asked.

She continued, "So many fish in the sea," and "Phish is the band for me" and "those phishing schemes ain't got integrity."

"Nice rhymes," I said.

She was obviously manic. She sounded like a Dr. Seuss book with her "clang" and had a "flight of ideas," bouncing from one subject to the next. It was clear she hadn't slept all night, and unlike me, didn't feel she needed the sleep.

"Where were you tonight?" I asked, yawning.

"Had to party, had to work, had to twerk," she said, as she started twerking. Her moves were good. She made me laugh. I liked her immediately.

"Drugs?" I asked. I was having trouble formulating full sentences.

"A beer for me, a beer for you, but don't do drugs, don't be a foo'," she said. Long story short, after a prolonged and labored exchange, she said she drank two beers but never did drugs.

She just kept talking. Talking and talking and talking. Her voice was so loud, and I had the worst headache. Please stop talking, I thought. Her mouth was on a motor. I could barely get a word in edgewise. My head was pounding, and it seemed like the fluorescent lights overhead had somehow gotten brighter than ever before.

"How'd you get here?" I asked. "Security didn't want to see my titties. They said insanity, but it don't have that gravity," she said.

It took me a while to figure out that she was talking about her hospitalization a few days ago for her first manic episode. I was scanning the medical records she brought with her as she danced and rhymed.

She was a college freshman who was depressed in high school but never manic before now. She was diagnosed with bipolar disorder after spending $10,000 in a casino, ripping her shirt off, and standing on the craps table asking who wanted to "have a go." Luckily, the only one to respond was a security officer, who had the sense to call an ambulance rather than the police.

The papers said she quickly stabilized and was never dangerous or suicidal. No mention of her family was made, which would generally concern me for a 19-year-old, but I was so tired it didn't register. I was thrilled that she was on good medications and had a psychiatrist appointment in 2 days. There didn't seem to be any imminent danger or reason to try to hospitalize her.

"Can I call your parents?" I asked.

"Mom's in Asia on a business trip and dad's a dick," she said. "And a prick. He don't care that I'm sick."

She denied suicidal or homicidal thoughts and didn't seem psychotic. Still, manic patients can ruin their lives from sheer impulsivity—in a day, you can write a nasty email to a boss or professor, blow through your bank account, and cheat on your partner.

Was she taking risks? Spending money? Having promiscuous sex? Taking on odd projects that would get her in trouble? She said no, so it seemed hard to justify an emergency worthy of breaking HIPAA privacy laws to call her parents against her will. Usually, I would have pushed harder, but all I could think about was sleep.

"Why did you come here, again?" I asked 30 minutes into the interview, confused, but I didn't even wait for the answer before asking, "Want to go home?"

She agreed, saying, "Doesn't matter anymore. It's all a bore. Sure, sure, sure."

I was confused. My thinking was foggy. I went to the staff room, rubbing my eyes, and asked the crisis counselor, "Why is she here, again?"

"Who knows," he said. "Probably bored. Send her home?"

I nodded, but was distracted by my clipboard. There was a Post-it Note in Spanish. How odd, I thought. I don't even speak Spanish. I stood there for a moment, marveling at my newfound linguistic abilities. "Whatchya doing, doc?" the crisis counselor asked.

"Do you know what this means?" I asked, handing him the note. I was so tired that I basically felt drunk.

"It's the list of Spanish TV shows I gave you when you said you liked *Narcos*," he said. "Go get some rest, doc."

I went back to the call room and fell into bed for somewhere between 2 and 20 minutes when the phone rang again.

"Avivia's dad on the line," the crisis counselor said. "Sounds upset. Patching him through."

"I'm looking for my daughter," he said. "Can you help me?"

I explained that I couldn't confirm or deny if I had seen her since I can't release information without a patient's consent, but I could take information.

"She's been missing for four days," he continued. "The college doesn't know where she is, her friends don't know, and her phone is off."

Clearly, no one called him from the hospital. He went on, sounding panicked, "She left me a voicemail a few hours ago saying 'goodbye and fuck you.' She said she's going to kill herself by walking in front of a train tonight. I called the police and five hospitals, but no one will help me. I don't know what to do."

My heart sank. Maybe she just wanted attention or was being provocative, I hoped. Maybe she said things like this to her dad because she hated him and wanted to worry him. I asked, "Has she said things like that before?"

"Never," he said. I could hear him crying on the other end of the line.

Fuck, I thought. I had made a technically correct decision that was totally wrong. I felt like anything that befell her would be my fault. She had obvious risk factors for suicide: bipolar disorder, recent discharge from an inpatient unit, and alcohol in her bloodstream. I should have dug deeper. I should have pushed her harder for information. I should have called her parents without her permission.

I put him on hold and sprinted down the hall, hoping to intercept her before she was discharged.

"Where is she?" I asked security, out of breath.

"Gone," they said. "Just left. You discharged her, didn't you?"

"I gotta get her," I said. "Unlock the door." She wasn't my patient anymore. If I started an involuntary petition and called it into the police, it might take them hours or days to find her and bring her back to the ER. She could be missing or dead by then.

"You gonna chase a patient in the street, doc? We don't do that," the security officer said. "They come to us."

"Let me out," I said.

As soon as I reached the pavement, I saw her in the distance, walking towards the rising sun, vaguely in the direction of the train tracks. I ran. In half a block, I tripped on my scrub pants, which were way too long, and fell. My pants were ripped, and my palms were bleeding by the time I caught up to her, out of breath.

"Wait!" I shouted. "I made a mistake. I shouldn't have let you leave." She shrugged and kept walking. I followed her.

"I haven't slept more than three hours straight in a week. You know what that's like, right? I'm not thinking straight. I didn't hear what you were trying to tell me. Probably, no one has," I continued.

Her face looked blank, unmoved, and she kept walking. I stood still and did something you're never supposed to do in front of patients: I cried. Not a few tears, but full, loud, uncontrollable sobbing she could easily hear down the block. It was sudden and unexpected, like a floodgate opening. I slumped against a brick wall, thinking I had just signed her death warrant and there was nothing I could do.

She wandered back to me and asked, "You okay?"

"Give me another chance!" I said, trying to wipe away the tears and catch my breath. "Please, please, give me another chance. I'll never forgive myself if something happens to you tonight."

If anyone saw us, they would definitely have thought I was the patient, crying and disheveled, collapsed against a brick wall while she stood above me, well dressed and now calm.

"It's okay, lady psychiatrist queen," she said, "I'll go with you." She reached out her hand to help me up off the ground and led me back to the ER.

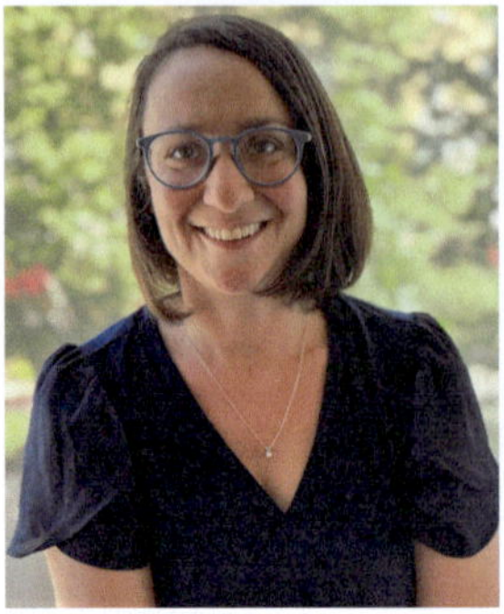

Dr. Lisa Jacobs is a child, adolescent, and adult psychiatrist in private practice in New York City and New Jersey. She serves as an Adjunct Clinical Assistant Professor in the Department of Psychiatry & Behavioral Sciences of the Stanford University School of Medicine. She serves as a group leader in The Pegasus Physician Writers at Stanford. She graduated from Cornell University and completed her medical training at Brown University, The University of Pennsylvania, and Stanford University. She is the 2019 winner in the prose category of the Irvin D. Yalom Literary Award for her short story, "Trapped in a Blizzard with a Politician in Withdrawal."

8 A Medical School Curse

Allison Neeson

During the gastrointestinal block of medical school, my cousin stopped eating. He was ten and absolutely refused to speak about it. We sought out therapists, doctors, teachers, and finally, after many tears and coaxing, an endoscopic biopsy. As a first-year medical student eager to share my thoughts, I offered a diagnosis: eosinophilic esophagitis. There had been a lecture on this esophageal allergy just that week, and admittedly, it was the only pediatric GI disease I knew. Inexplicably, I was right.

A pattern emerged.

During the Rheumatology course, a friend's mom got her shoulder replaced, and we discussed the physiology of osteoarthritis over dinner. When my boyfriend's dad had Bell's Palsy during Neurology, I consulted the lecture slides on how to distinguish stroke from the significantly less scary nerve problem, as I gathered his physical exam over FaceTime.

With every block of our curriculum, a condition from class seemed to magically materialize in someone I knew. Had my friends and family always gotten so many weird illnesses? I considered the availability bias, knowing that simply learning about

A. Neeson (✉)
Department of Pediatrics, Children's Hospital of Philadelphia, Philadelphia, PA, USA
e-mail: neesona@chop.edu

J. Pien et al. (eds.), *Onward*,
https://doi.org/10.1007/978-3-032-15776-8_8

the pathologies might make me notice them more. I tried not to fall victim to medical student hypochondriasis, but I began to think I might be cursed.

Still, these lecture-slides-turned-medical-realities were innocuous enough. It became a joke amongst my friends, speculating which disease would come alive next. And despite the minor anxieties the curse aroused (I was very on edge during the Reproductive block, when I found myself, "a previously healthy 24-year-old female," in the stem of every question), the opportunity to test my diagnostic abilities was even fun. But it was a curse, after all, and it was only a matter of time until malediction turned malady.

The cancer came early, three blocks before the Oncology course. It came during the Respiratory unit, though it was gastrointestinal in nature.

My grandmother's original cholecystectomy had been cancelled at the beginning of the pandemic, when elective surgeries were halted. Then her gallstones became emergent, several weeks and many more COVID cases later, and she found herself checking into a COVID-filled emergency room. My frustration that she couldn't have the surgery as originally scheduled, when the risk of exposure to the virus was much lower, was validated when she received a positive test for the coronavirus a few days after her hospital stay. In exchange for her gallbladder, they gave her COVID-19. But the worst news came from the first-year resident who saw my grandmother after the surgery.

"The surgery went well, but they are taking the gallbladder to pathology because it looked abnormal. It could be cancer."

She is nonchalant and mildly in a rush. She leaves my grandmother alone. Cancer? It's a pandemic, and there are no visitors allowed. I imagine my grandmother in a hospital room by herself, absorbing this news. Her aloneness sounds isolating, but I think she might have appreciated the solitude—a welcome respite from the relative chaos of our home, full of grandchildren and parents and cats.

I grew up in my grandmother's house, where I had a beautiful childhood. We call grandma "Momom," an apt title for a grandmother who often felt more like a second mom. Still, between her second-mom tasks of car-pooling and back-to-school shopping, Momom succumbed to her grandmotherly instinct to dote on her grandchildren profusely. There was always a silly story to be told, made-up while we snuggled under her comforter, a pool to float around in our backyard, daring each other to brave the deep end (the alleged home of Jabba the Hutt; though never proven, *I* certainly wasn't going to risk finding out). Momom dutifully revealed the back side of my flashcards through high school, indulged the neon green wall color I requested for my bedroom as a pre-teen, and ensured robust evidence of Santa's existence with a family room full of presents every Christmas.

When my friends found out my grandmother had COVID-19, they were worried in a way I couldn't bring myself to be. I thought: Who cares if she has COVID? She's going to die of cancer. I couldn't worry because worrying meant acknowledging her mortality, and I had long ago decided that grandmothers are invincible. I couldn't worry because I needed to Google things. My family had questions, and I, the first-year medical student, was supposed to find the answers. While she suffered through pneumonia, I learned how blood cells trade carbon dioxide for oxygen in our lungs, texting my mom between classes to assess Momom's oxygen saturation. It dropped, but never too much. Thankfully, she avoided the worst symptoms of the coronavirus and was able to recover. With her recovery came a false sense of relief. My family was eager for her to begin her cancer treatment, so she could recover from that, too. Now, I was worried in a way they didn't realize they should be.

In the first few days of my grandmother's cancer diagnosis, my mom asked me what I knew about gallbladder cancer. I had already read the single PowerPoint slide on gallbladder neoplasia from the "GI cancers" lecture dozens of times. It is mostly empty, and says:

- In <1% of patients with gallstones
- Most discovered late
- Overall 5-year survival: 5–12%

I told her we hadn't learned about it.

My grandmother, however, is not so naïve. An emergency room nurse for decades and then in the homes of permanently disabled children, Momom knows suffering.

"I've been reading online. The prognosis is terrible," she said to me on a recent phone call.

I considered how to respond, thinking about the woman who is the most important influence in my life. The reason I am in medical school, the reason I love to read, and why I crave chicken and dumpling soup when I am sick. Is she asking me as a medical student or as a granddaughter?

"It's not as bad as you think," I replied.

I chose to respond as a granddaughter, though I wondered how different my medical student response would have been. I think the prognosis is bad, but maybe she thinks it's *worse*, I justified to myself. What good does it do to scare her? I could rationalize the lie under the guise of "doing no harm." It felt kinder to protect her from the worry that I feel. Really, it was kinder to me, too afraid to say what is hard. I recognize this cowardice, yet I have to wonder: where is the line between lying and being hopeful? Isn't there healing to be found in optimism?

We're taught that everything a doctor does, even the way a surgeon walks out of the operating room, can confer a placebo effect, bolstering recovery. I think again about the intern, the first doctor to introduce the cancer to my grandmother. Did she practice what she was going to say before she went into the room? I think about Momom, in the moments after she received the news but before she told us, when the diagnosis was only hers to hold. Who will take care of them? I imagine she wondered.

And it's true. Who do I call when I need to befriend the nurses on clinical rotations and don't know how? Who will make sure my roommates have phone-banked enough in the next election to meet her standard for people I am allowed to live with? Does anyone even know where the chicken and dumpling soup recipe is written down? Not to mention what stories to tell under worn-in-comforters and how to know what integrity and grit and selflessness look like. What happens to all of her books, and the ones I will never get to recommend?

Our next block is called “Disaster Medicine.” Last year, I would have feared what the med-school curse had in store. But my disaster in medicine has already happened, and the bullet point that says, “5% overall 5-year survival” has remained clear for every unit since. I see it in board review materials, when my throat tightens at the flashcard for Capecitabine, thinking about the blisters it causes on her feet. I hear it in the patient history, given by a grandmother, here with her grandson, at the pediatrician’s office where I work this semester. I feel it in the silence after our phone calls end and in the decision to travel or not travel home to see her for Christmas this year.

I know my med-school curse has plagued many medical students before me. I take comfort in the collectivity of it: everyone who practices medicine is also a patient, mother, friend, and granddaughter. It is a difficult role to play, simultaneously a medical informant and a regular, grieving human. I don’t feel obligated by anyone to perfect the balance of these identities, nor do I resent the occasional burden they inflict on each other. Though my grief sometimes makes studying hard, I take pride in my unique position as a medical-student-granddaughter. I can provide information, interpret labs and scans and translate doctor-jargon into a comprehensible language my family can digest. I am more motivated than ever to learn, excited to understand the physiology, knowing it will enable me to explain pathologies to families and patients, as I do to my own family now. I know embracing these dual roles will make me a better physician. In the meantime, I hope it will make me a better granddaughter, too.

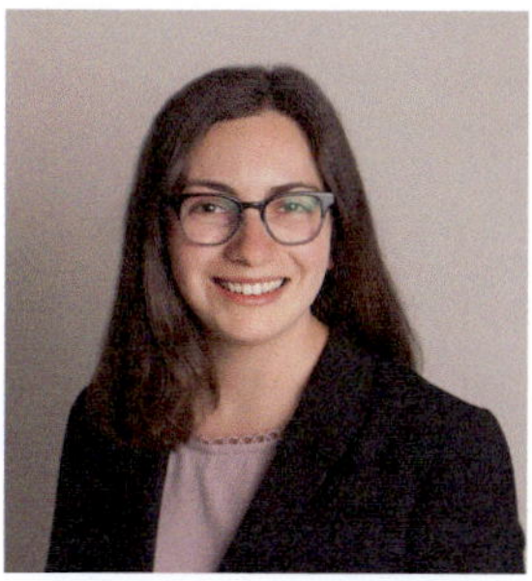

Allison Neeson is a Pediatrics Resident at the Children’s Hospital of Philadelphia in the Leadership in Equity, Advocacy, and Policy track.

9 Deep Love

Ava Satnick

Grief stabbed and tore through my chest as deep and immense as the open seas. My joints stiffened with corrugated glass. A tight band wrapped around my torso prevented me from breathing. The heaviness of my limply held limbs brought me to my knees, suffocating me in mourning.

My phone rang at 7:30am in the morning. It was January 3. Outside was a frigid 28 degrees. I turned over in bed to pick up my cell phone off the windowsill near my head—a space-saving trick I learned in my cozy 500 square foot New York City apartment. From October to February, the apartment overheated, and I left the window open a crack, exposing the chilled air and an inch of snow. The phone was cold in my hands. I was a pediatrician in a private practice then, and it was not an unusual time for a patient to call right before the office opened. I checked the screen.

Caller ID read: Daniel. A picture of his glistening forehead shone through on the screen.

It still shocked me to see my baby brother bald. He didn't have to speak because I knew what he was going to say. Dad died last night in his sleep.

A different call in a different season of a different morning came through to me 9 months prior. It was spring in the city, the cherry blossoms were blooming, and spring fever was aris-

A. Satnick (✉)
Stanford University School of Medicine, Stanford, CA, USA

J. Pien et al. (eds.), *Onward*,
https://doi.org/10.1007/978-3-032-15776-8_9

ing in the streets of New York City. "Mom fell while riding her bike and hit the ground so hard the bike bent in half and her helmet shattered." My father, Steve, had called me with this startling news after getting word from a neighbor. "Steve, your wife has been taken by ambulance," echoed the neighbor's voice intended to catch my father's attention on the home answering machine.

A CT scan was ordered. My father's voice sounded hollow and shaky when he told me. It was soon drowned out by alarms blaring in the background. I had a sigh of relief knowing no fatal bleed would wait for a final read. He must not be thinking straight and may be hypoglycemic from his morning routine. Two cups of coffee before 6 AM, the New York Times crossword puzzle, and off to the gym. He would spend 2 hours there alternating between the treadmill, elliptical, weights, and swimming. He called this his physical therapy, which he self-prescribed, to treat his idiopathic peripheral neuropathy. He received the diagnosis when he was only 37 years old. It must have been an interesting time then: my brother was losing his baby teeth, I was overcoming my fear of Mickey, and dad was relearning how to walk without feeling in his feet.

As kids, my brother and I would play doctor in the back seat on the weekly trip to visit our cousins for dinner.

"Beep, beep, beep," went the pager.

We would pull over and then out came the 1990s Nokia cell phone.

"Hi, it's Dr. Satnick, returning a call," he'd say, our cue for silence as my father, the allergist, took down the chief complaint, and we would try to guess it: wheezing, running nose, or coughing fit.

We were clued in by dad's follow-up questions: "For how long? What was the trigger?

How many breaths per minute?"

It's a toss-up if my younger brother's first word was "fried rice" or "prednisone." Both were commonly ordered then, along with wonton soups and shrimp with black bean sauce for the table seating 10 with a central lazy Susan.

When I arrived at the hospital to visit my mom, my father was moving up and down the corridors like an antelope on a log. His chronic condition stole his lower extremity proprioception. I had grown accustomed to his gait. I did not notice when his left calf atrophied or his shins had pitting edema. It was normal when he was at home self-infusing IV-IG, and sometimes I helped. My most vivid memories of childhood involved swimming laps on Sunday morning, the smell of his homemade French Toast on Saturdays, and learning how to do a venipuncture on Friday evenings. I was surprised when on my first attempt in medical school, I gave my classmate a hematoma.

"It's much easier to do this on my dad's veins," I said.

I was glad I stopped to pick up a sandwich before going to the hospital.

"Roast beef on a hero. Hold the tomatoes. My father does not like soggy bread," I reminded the deli-man who had served us since I was a kid.

At the foot of my mother's hospital bed, my father was a second away from eating his hand. He often ate when he was nervous or stressed. Many late nights, I would find him passed out on the couch in the den with popcorn kernels or pie on his chest, rising and falling with each breath. Having a condition that prevented him from activity threatened his identity as a fit man. Gone were his days of dancing, but I kept my memories of twirling to Broadway soundtracks or Smokey Joe's Cafe on replay.

He finished his sandwich and took out his phone to update my aunt. He said, "We are waiting for the results of her CT scan."

I was with my father when the results of my mom's CT scan came back. No internal bleeding. It was just a concussion. The expectation was full recovery. Within a few hours, she was regaining her memory and speech. My father and I shared a chuckle when my mother looked at me and said, "Did you clean out your closets yet?" Organization is her love language.

My father's tests had always been inconclusive. The lab draws, lumbar punctures, and MRI scans did not elucidate answers for why he felt numbness and stabbing pain from his toes to his knees. Doctors, medicines, and procedures could not cure him. He had to carry his pain everywhere he went. Peripheral neuropathy caused the constant feeling of pins and needles in his legs: during my soccer games, graduations, at the beach, at the dinner table, in the office seeing patients. Despite the pain and depression, he was known for his boisterous laugh, caring for others, and gregarious energy.

Feeling relieved, my father left the bedside to update the family. I waited and then followed him. Down the hospital corridors we went, between the hollow, ashen-yellow walls, fluorescent lights, and a sign that read "EMPLOYEES" in red. I heard his voice steady as he said three words I will never forget, with composure from his vagus nerve and diaphragm, "Ava is here."

Those were the last few words of impact I remember he said. In that cold winter January morning my brother called me to announce our father's death. I carried my grief everywhere I went. At first, it was gushing, predictable, and constant. I must have cried enough tears to extinguish wildfires, I was moving to California then. I canceled my attendance at weddings, celebrations, and anything happy. To work, I went braless, then part-time, and then I had to quit.

Grief became my job. It did not provide holidays, lunch hours, or benefits. Strangers would console me wherever I was sobbing: online for groceries, on the subway, or wailing on all fours in the locker room at the gym in nothing but a towel to cover my feeling of brokenness.

A woman looked at me in awe and said, "I never loved someone as deeply."

When my brother called in January, my worldview turned upside down. Ten days later in Patagonia, at the apex of El Capitan, I could not have been further away from my childhood dreamland. The wind stilled, and I could hear those three words again. "Ava is here." And in that moment, I also realized how important I was to him. My father was never one to like too much doting or attention, and after a moment passed, I could hear him add, "Now go back and join your friends." On that mountain apex, I began a life with a whole new perspective.

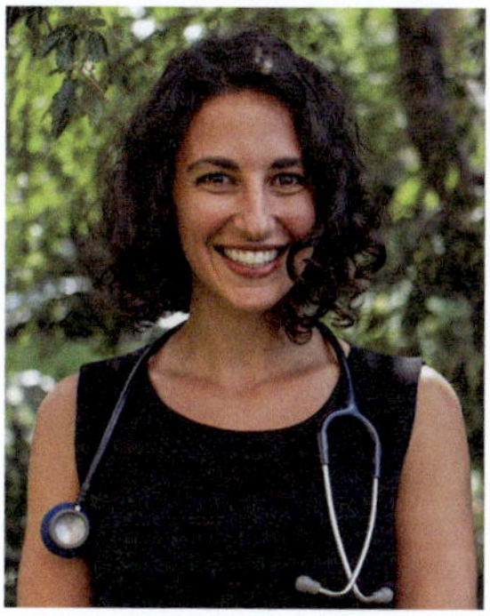

Ava Satnick, MD, is a board-certified pediatrician and native New Yorker who moved across the country to pursue integrative medicine training at Stanford University in Palo Alto, California. While she thought she was moving to California to be trained by the best and brightest integrative medicine physicians in the country, (which she was), she also learned the art of healing from her own personal experience. Six months before her planned departure to the west coast her father, also a physician, suddenly passed overnight. When she arrived in California, she was in a state of immense shock and grief. Through her own experiences and work with physician mentors, various healing modalities and practitioners, and her community, she arrived at a much deeper appreciation for integrative medicine, and self healing than she could have learned in textbooks and reading. In the height of the 2020 coronavirus pandemic, she began her own practice in Portola Valley, California, where she used what she has learned from both clinical training and personal experience to help others along their journeys to achieve joyous living. The name of her practice, Holbrook Health from 202-2025, is in honor of her father whose office was in a town called Holbrook, New York. When he awoke every morning he would say he was "off to Holbrook," and then she too can say that anywhere she is in the world offering virtual and in person consultations. Her current passion is facilitating workshops and retreats and coaching for physicians or healthcare providers who have gone through burnout themselves. To stay up to date you can reach her at (650)422-1143 or avasatnick@gmail.com.

Shadow 10

Jennifer Soh

It's 5:45 am when I jump out of bed at the sound of my alarm and scramble to quiet the incessant beeping before it wakes my roommate. She stirs in her corner of the room before slipping back into a state of deep sleep. She'll stay there, like the rest of campus, for at least a couple more hours. If it wasn't for the combination of excitement and nerves sending excessive amounts of adrenaline through my body, I would join everyone and crawl back into the comfort of my bed.

Instead, I quickly brush my teeth in the dark and throw on dress pants for professionalism, sneakers for comfort, and a collared short-sleeve shirt for infection prevention. There's no time to eat anything before I run down four flights of stairs and into the parking garage.

It's my first time navigating the road to the university hospital. It's also my first time driving this early in the morning. There's this familiar, eerie loneliness to the car ride, though. The premed years have no shortage of packed lecture halls or classmates to commiserate with, but the weekends spent locked in study rooms and 10-minute meals scarfing down dinner alone before chemistry office hours can't help but feel isolating. For the first time, the rest of the world feels just as lonely as I do. The sky is a piercing shade

J. Soh (✉)
Stanford University, Stanford, USA

J. Pien et al. (eds.), *Onward*,
https://doi.org/10.1007/978-3-032-15776-8_10

of dark and the shopping center that sits across the street from the front entrance of the children's hospital is empty.

Even amidst all this stillness, the sliding doors to the hospital continue to open and close. The contrast between the two is so striking. It feels almost ironic that in just a few hours, someone will be browsing the aisles of The Container Store while in the building next door, another person will be dying.

As soon as I make it inside the hospital, I'm greeted by a security guard who sees the presence of a badge clipped onto my shirt and nods hello. There are a couple other people in the lobby who look like family members of a patient. I watch them play an intricate waiting game—two laps around the chairs, sitting for two seconds, then two more laps—while I debate with myself if I should take a seat or stay standing. The more I debate, the more anxious I feel that I am not in the right lobby or I somehow got the date wrong. I start drafting a text to Taylor, the resident who I'm shadowing for the day. "Hi, I'm here!" feels too casual, but "Hello, I just got to the lobby and wanted to make sure I'm in the right place" feels like I'm being passive-aggressive that she's late. I try adding some exclamation points and a tasteful emoji when someone in blue scrubs who looks like she could be a third-year pediatric resident comes rushing through the front door.

"Hi, I'm Taylor," she says.

"Hi Taylor, thank you so much for –" I start. She grabs her phone that already has a life of its own, buzzing with questions and ringing with orders. She starts walking in the middle of my sentence, so I turn my focus to walking behind her instead, each one of my steps matching where hers just left off. Like a shadow.

Taylor leads me through a maze of green and purple corridors and doors. I blindly follow through a series of rights and lefts, two flights of stairs, and a handwashing station. We end at a door labeled "STAFF ONLY" in bright, red letters. There's one other person in the room who greets Taylor with a sigh.

"You're going to have one long day," he says. It makes her chuckle, so I feel the need to smile too. The tips of his otherwise black hair are bleached yellow. There's an empty, crushed can of Monster Energy at his desk.

"You're an undergrad?" He asks, noticing my badge. I nod.

"Um, yeah—yes. Taylor is letting me shadow her –"He cuts off the rest of my sentence. I guess it's normal to do this here.

"Don't do it." It comes out of nowhere. I think he might be joking, but his face doesn't change—the corners of his lips remain downturned, and his eyes are stoic.

"It?" I'm taken aback.

"You might think you're different." He turns his attention back to his computer, scrolling through charts of numbers and shaking his head. "You might think you want it more than everyone else. But then you're gonna be me, wishing at two in the morning you did literally anything else with your life."

What a welcome.

I want to be a doctor. Badly. So much so that no class or exam or late night or early morning during my first two years of college has ever made me think differently. I watched classmates leave with each chemistry class we trudged through. For others, it took having to cut into a cadaver during anatomy lab to realize that medicine wasn't the life they wanted. But I've stayed. Maybe I do think that I want it more.

I don't quite know how to respond, so I open my mouth and hope something eloquent, or at least reasonable, comes out.

"Oh, I –"

"Shut up, don't scare her." Taylor smacks him on the shoulder. "Don't listen to anyone after they're on nights. And it's just residency. Life supposedly gets better after it." He scoffs, rattles off a few names and scary-sounding words, then leaves to go home for the first time in 12 hours.

Taylor sits me down on a half-broken chair next to her desk and begins clicking through the chart of a 2-month-old boy with Apert Syndrome and imminent lung failure.

"Ugh, he looks worse." Taylor groans. I don't quite know what Apert Syndrome is or which one of the tiny numbers on her screen she's referring to. But I feel like my presence alone is already enough of a bother for Taylor today, so I just nod and try to make myself as small as possible on the chair. As if that makes me less of a burden.

We continue like this. Taylor, muttering to herself, explaining a condition here and there or how the PICU is sort of also functioning as the NICU this week because of residual overflow from a MRSA outbreak in the actual NICU, or how today's attending is known for impossible pimp questions, which is not only nerve-wracking but also incredibly inconvenient and annoying. I keep nodding periodically through it all. I'm too scared to ask any questions. I know too little about medicine or hospitals to gauge if they're good questions or not. So, I stay quiet instead.

"Rounds," Taylor says. "Let's go." She doesn't need to say "stand to the side" or "don't get in the way" for me to know that I should continue making myself take up as little space as possible.

We head down the hall and join the group of two other residents, one fellow, and the infamous attending. I can hear our first stop before I can see it. As soon as we turn the corner and into a bay of infants, an ear-splitting wail bounces off the walls.

"That would be Luis – scratch that, Frederick. There's a story there." Taylor pulls out a folded sheet of paper from the back pocket of her scrubs. "Two-week-old baby boy, here due to opioid withdrawal." Luis, or Frederick, is the smallest baby I have ever seen. His cheeks are bright red from screaming, and I can see small beads of sweat pooling around his nose. I watch his hands clench themselves into balls. His legs and arms thrash while Taylor and the attending go back and forth about morphine dosages. Once the nurse administers some through his tiny IV, his screams slow to a stop. The shock from the initial mention of opioid withdrawal is drowned out by the shock of seeing a baby so tiny receive morphine.

"So what's the story about the name?" the attending finally asks.

"Oh, right. So mom had cardiovascular complications during delivery, so she's been in the cardio unit herself. I've been calling to keep her updated on baby boy, and I kept referring to him as Luis because that's what's on his birth certificate. She sounded confused when I called her yesterday and kept insisting that his name is Frederick." Taylor shrugs.

"Frederick it is," the attending says, matter-of-factly. "What's the mom's story?"

"When the social worker first asked her, she denied any drug use, but with Lui—Frederick's symptoms, she told us she used heroin 2–3 times during the pregnancy."

"Any other family we know of?"

Taylor shakes her head.

"Did we call CPS?"

"CPS has been called, and the social worker should be coming in later. I can update them again, too."

"Alrighty then." With that, the attending leaves Frederick's bed, and the rest of the group trails behind. The back-and-forth nature of the conversation makes me feel like it's just another day at the office for everyone but me. No one else seems to share my shock, let alone my horror. The team just moves on. One of the other residents prepares to present the next patient. A second-year resident leans over to whisper to Taylor.

"I mean, my question is, why only 2–3 times?!" It's meant to be a joke. It paralyzes me. The two of them chuckle together.

There's a sudden onset of nausea that washes over me. I can't tell if it's happening because I haven't eaten or had anything to drink all morning, or if it was from this new feeling of disgust that I can't shake. Frederick's screams, the fact that his mother doesn't know his name, how he needs morphine to live—I want to scream. This situation being construed into a joke is unfathomable to me. The fact that it was made into one is the biggest shock of all.

We make it to Ana, a 5-month-old baby girl who is nestled in the arms of her mother. I can't see her face, but the top of her head could look relatively healthy if I just ignore the tangled mess of wires and tubes feeding in and out of her. There's a whiteboard in the corner of her room—Name: Ana, Weight: 4.8 kg, Height: 56 cm, I need: diapers.

"She's had too many scans since she was born, do we really need to do another one?" Her mother is exasperated. I can tell how hard she's trying to not raise her voice while Ana is sleeping. Her exasperation doesn't change the rhythmic cadence of her knees, bending and extending and bending and extending.

"If it can be avoided, we would like for you not to do it." Ana's dad is much taller than anyone else in the room. His voice is stern and rough.

"We understand, but you want answers, and we're trying to give them to you." The conversation continues until it sounds like an argument. I'm not entirely sure what the argument is about.

The attending has the last say. I follow the team out of the room, shutting the door behind me. He shakes his head.

"I mean they're counting how many scans she's had since the day she was born," he mutters. The rest of the team nods.

"Quite particular people, aren't they?" he says. I watch the first-year resident mark Ana's name on her printed sheet of notes. She scribbles, "Difficult parents," using her hand as a flat surface to write.

The language they're using to describe the interaction stuns me. Where in the years of training, exams, rotations, overnight shifts, cross-country moves, long-distance relationships, missed birthdays and holidays, all the guilt, the doubt, the stress, and the worry during the training it takes to become a doctor does a person break and "rightfully concerned parents" turn into "difficult," "particular" ones?

It feels unreasonable to me. I find it hard to believe that I'm the only one who feels this way, but everyone seems unfazed by the interaction and the conversation that followed. I tell myself to get over it. I convince myself that maybe I'm the unreasonable one. After all, what do I know?

And so, with the rest of the team, I move on.

Adrian's room is next. Adrian is a 7-month-old baby boy with a congenital heart defect. He is in his bed alone. Two other people are in the room during his presentation, sitting quietly at the windowsill with their hands in their laps. One looks like she is in elementary school, maybe middle school at best. I think the other is Adrian's mother.

The team talks in front of the two, rather than with them, quickly coming to a consensus about the next steps in Adrian's care plan. We all leave the room without acknowledging the two other people in the room again. Once his doors are closed, Taylor stays back to talk to me.

"Remember that girl in the windowsill? The one with the *My Little Pony* shirt?"

"Yeah," I respond, confused as to what could be so pressing that Taylor was missing the beginning of the next patient's presentation for.

"That's Adrian's mother. She's 12." I let a *woah* escape from my lips because I have no other words. I try to keep up with Taylor's quick strides. My brain can't help but do the math to count the 7 months of Adrian's life and 9 months of pregnancy that should be subtracted from her current age.

"I know. The situation is… awkward." Taylor sprints to meet the rest of the team, leaving me to move and process this information more slowly. The feeling of nausea hasn't left me this entire time. I begin to realize that it's a manifestation of guilt. I had been so excited to come into the hospital today. The gravity of what that means hits me. I had been so excited to see this.

This isn't awkward. This is devastating and painful and horrifying.

I don't even listen to the next few patients. I can't take it anymore. But everyone moves on to the next patient. Then, the next. And the next.

After two and a half hours of rounds, we come to our last patient.

"We always save her for last," Taylor says. Before I ask why, I step into her room to find that her walls are empty, void of any pictures or decor like the other patients'. The visitor's chairs are empty too. Evie is in the middle of the bed, quiet. Her nurse has braided the tufts of her curls together. *Paw Patrol* is playing on the television in front of her, but she doesn't seem to be watching it. The cartoon animals bounce right off of her pupils instead.

The only thing that I can understand from Taylor's presentation is that Evie is slowly dying. The cardiology, pulmonology, and neurology teams will be up to talk to the rest of the team, but no one wants to take responsibility for her. Taylor explains that her parents live in Sacramento and can't make the trip to visit her often. So, Evie has been slowly dying in this room, alone.

My chest had been feeling heavier and heavier with each patient. Now it feels like a rock has been dropped on it and is squeezing the rest of the oxygen out of my lungs.

"We'll hold her Goals of Care meeting over Zoom at noon with the parents. I imagine they'll have a lot of questions about her condition because they haven't seen her in a couple of weeks. I think they still had a lot of hope left from when they last visited," Taylor says. Is it wrong to hope that a parent has given up on their child's life? Would that make this conversation any easier?

"Have we tried transferring her?" The attending asks.

"No one wants to take her." Taylor says it like it is a simple fact. The rest of the team just accepts it. There was nothing more to do, so we leave Evie's room. I wave bye to Evie as I walk past her bed to the door. I don't know why I do it.

The team disperses to finish writing up orders and documenting the past three hours into sparse sentences. Taylor's phone starts to receive texts from the pharmacists and respiratory therapists and nurses. She walks and answers them. I follow.

"So the Goals of Care meeting is where we'll discuss with the parents about what they hope we can prioritize for Evie. But I don't think there's a lot of time left for her, so that's probably what we're going to talk about. You're welcome to join it at –"

"I'm so sorry, I actually have a meeting, so I might need to leave soon." We had planned for me to stay the whole day, so I share Taylor's confusion as to why I just blurted out a very swift, very untrue departure. But the thought of hearing her explain to Evie's parents that there is nothing more she can medically do for their dying daughter is more than I can handle today.

No textbook or lecture could have ever prepared me for this type of grief. In a couple of weeks, this beautiful girl will be gone.

"Oh, no worries. Yeah, feel free to leave whenever you need to." I want to ask if Taylor feels the same way I do. I want to ask if the fact that I've been on the verge of tears all morning means that I'm not cut out for this. I want to ask if this is really what being a doctor is like and what happens if I can't move on like everyone else can. Instead, all I say is, "Thank you, again. I, um, learned so much." Taylor nods and returns to her phone.

I feel sick. I can't help but wish I had crawled back into bed when I still had the chance. I grab my backpack from the workroom and try to find my way out of the maze of green and purple corridors and doors to the front entrance as fast as I can, as if the faster I move, the faster I can outrun all of the guilt and the horror and the pain of the morning.

The sun has been out for hours. The parking lot at The Container Store is now full. I start grabbing as much fresh, vibrant air as I can. I force it all into my lungs in huge, greedy gulps. Once I make it to the seat of my car, I finally let myself cry. For Frederick, for Ana, for Adrian, and for Evie.

I cry for myself last.

*Note: Names and any other identifying information have been changed for anonymity.

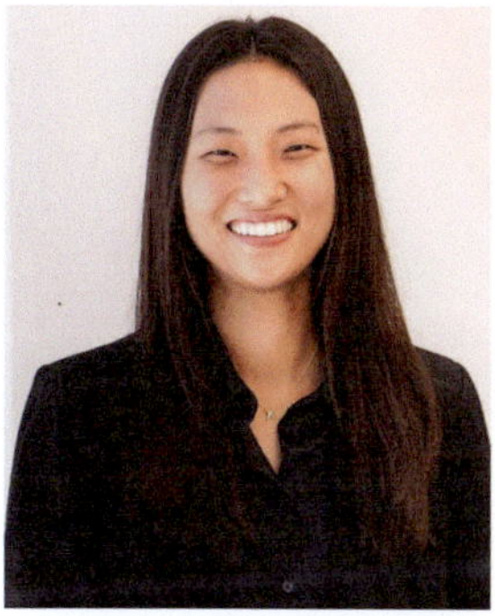

Jennifer Soh received a master's degree from Stanford Medicine in Community Health and Prevention Research and a bachelor's degree from Stanford University in Bioengineering. She has been an active member of the Pegasus Physician Writers since 2021. She hopes to pursue a career working with underserved communities and writing to uplift and reflect on community stories.

11 The Return of the Night Visitor

Hans Steiner and Lisa Jacobs

A hard knock on my door. I cracked it open and said, "I am in a meeting."

"Henry says he has to talk to you right now".

I excused myself and picked up the line in another office. Henry's voice sounded as if he was choking, or throwing up.

"I just got a letter from Mom. I am not sure what to do," he said.

It was not unusual for Henry to have problems with his parents. What was unusual was that he called for help.

"Can you come in and see me today?" I asked.

"I'm still in Santa Barbara. I have to finish a bunch of stuff," he explained.

"What does the letter say? Can you read it to me?"

Silence. Then I heard paper rustling.

"Henry, are you there?"

He started reading with a voice broken by tears, "When you read this, I will be dead."

I could not breathe, but tried to sound calm as I asked, "Where is she?"

I started seeing Henry when he was 16, at the request of his father, Oliver, a professor in the business school. Henry now was a 22-year-old

H. Steiner (✉) · L. Jacobs
Department of Psychiatry and Behavioral Sciences,
Stanford University School of Medicine, Stanford, CA, USA

J. Pien et al. (eds.), *Onward*,
https://doi.org/10.1007/978-3-032-15776-8_11

junior in college. Despite being a very intelligent young man, he managed to get mostly failing grades in high school. This drove Oliver crazy and into my office. Henry's mother, Charlette ("It rhymes with Scarlette," she would add), feebly agreed with her former husband, but I never got the sense that she was as concerned or invested in her son's academic progress as Oliver. She seemed too preoccupied with herself.

From the beginning, treatment did not progress as I had hoped. Both parents, for their own special reasons, struggled to provide the necessary presence for Henry, in therapy as well as at home. This showed up in Henry missing many sessions. True, early sessions with adolescents rarely flow. I was used to working hard to get them to disclose concerns and what was happening at home. Henry was, if anything, more extreme: he made me think of a medieval castle, drawbridge up, deep moat around the steep and rising walls, turrets with guards everywhere.

While Oliver had brought Henry for treatment, he was also a numbers man, expecting immediate results, akin to treating a strep infection with penicillin. Still, initially, he found some time to bring Henry and a long list of complaints about some aspect of academic performance.

"Henry, tell Hans, why you got a B minus on the math final." Turning to me, he added, "I know this kid, he is like me, he can crunch numbers with the best of them. Why the B minus?"

Before Henry could open his mouth, Oliver droned on about how all this had to change. Henry sat through these sermons, appearing contrite. But watching the emotional micro-expressions flickering across his face, I saw rage. At the end of the session, Oliver asked for a moment alone with me. Before I could say no, he pushed Henry out of the room and closed the door.

Getting serious, he confided, "Henry is too close to his mother, unable to man up. Hans, don't get me wrong: Charlette is hard to resist, charming to the point of being seductive with any man, and she makes no exception with Henry. Those Southern Beauties are all alike." Oliver pounded his right fist into his open palm: "Crewing and skippering on the San Francisco Bay is the antidote. I am willing to sacrifice myself for him. But you have to make him show up in school. You remember, Hans, I was raised in Connecticut. I love flying across rippled waters in sleek, fast 30 footers. Being a skipper is in my blood. Nothing better than sailing to teach how to take command."

Oliver jumped up, without waiting for my answer. "Well, we got this handled, right?"

He was gone before I could answer. In my next session alone with Henry, I returned to that moment.

"What do you think about what dad said last time?"

"I think he is right. But now I really will try harder. I am on top of it". As he said this, he looked as angry as when he talked to his father. Maybe there was a message to me, too: Lay off, you are pushing too hard. If so, Henry was unaware of it.

I decided to test the waters, saying, "Henry, let me tell you what I see. There is a loop that keeps repeating itself. He comes in with a list of problems, lectures you about them. When I stop him – not easy to do—and invite you to talk about your side of things, you quickly agree with him. It's like you are trying to silence me. But when he is talking, you look quite angry. Do you feel that at all?"

Henry looked surprised and said, "Angry? Not at all. He's got a point. He is the best dad. He just bought me my own sloop." A door barely opened was snapping shut.

What I was left with was the incongruence between what Henry said and what his emotions betrayed, like in a song where words and music don't go together. Henry was hiding behind a wall while making it look like he was working with me. Maybe shifting the discussion to mother would help.

"What's your mom say about all this school stuff?" I asked.

Henry chuckled. "This is confidential, right? No point getting her into trouble with dad. She doesn't even know the half of it. She is so into her own stuff. I barely see her. She is in her studio all the time. Or she is exhausted and sleeps."

Charlette confirmed Henry's account. She said she concentrated on her painting, being the life of any party, and getting plenty of sleep. She was an acclaimed artist with deep roots in the Garden District of New Orleans, 12 years younger than her husband. I rarely saw Charlette at any of Henry's appointments. Henry came either by train or caught a ride with a classmate, his sister, or neighbors. When I called to check into this, Charlette was very cordial and polite.

"There is always so much to do, doctor; you know what it's like. I truly am a single parent. I have all these shows going on, and vernissages. I'll try to get better about bringing him"

Talking to her felt like being wrapped up in a silken blanket. Her looks reminded me of Grace Kelly. She had golden hair, sparkling eyes, a soft voice, and a singsong accent.

At times, when I called her late in the afternoon or early in the evening to give her updates and request information, she would speak very slowly, saying, "I am dead tired, Doctor." I also noticed that sometimes she had no recall of what we had discussed just a couple days ago. I asked Henry about this.

"She sounds exhausted and loses the thread easily. Is she ok?" I asked. He responded.

Henry sat up straight in his chair. His face turned smooth and watchful. "Yes, of course." Henry reassured me that mother's malaise was not a problem. He just would do the cooking for the three of them, as he had been since the divorce. His sister would do the shopping, because she had a car. He liked it that Mom did not bug him about his homework, not like Dad. He liked his independence. It became clear that one of Henry's jobs was to protect mother, not make any demands, and be self-sufficient. That was his reality. Again, there was no opening. Henry was the man on the watchtower, the sentinel guardian of his family's secrets.

Oliver and Charlette divorced when Henry was 11, after his mother had yet another affair. Henry and his 17-year-old sister were to be raised by Charlette in a comfortable Hillsborough villa. But his father's firm had some "temporary cash flow problems," and he needed to sell the villa. He offered to move the family into a house in San Carlos. Shortly after the family moved, the cash flow stoppage was unplugged. Oliver earned millions having his company go public. He still sold the house in Hillsborough, but immediately invested in an 8000 square foot villa on the tip of Tiburon. As he said, he owed it to the children. However, the children remained in San Carlos. Oliver opined that children needed their mother.

Life in San Carlos was not as easy as it had been. The house on Arroyo Street was not far from El Camino Real, about 1,250 square feet on a 3,000 square feet lot, lots of traffic right nearby. The trip from San Carlos to the North Bay to visit Oliver was arduous, but he made it worth Henry's while: they sailed on the bay together. Henry joined a youth sailing club in Tiburon and made several friends, competing with them in races on the weekend.

Running into Henry's walls, moats, and watchtowers, not having his parents to help me break through, having a mother who was more concerned about the color combination of eye shadow and lipstick, and a father who was interested in Henry's "showing up and delivering" grades and sailing trophies often left me frustrated. Usually, I use this type of frustration to confront the patient and parents, but in Henry's case, I felt I had to be cautious, lest his avoidance turn into staying away. At best, I was a psychiatric cheering section. Trying to show him his rage about being deprived made no sense to him. But then, of course, there were his bad grades, a surefire way to keep the parents involved. These grades were driven by his unconscious rage. Without treating that dynamic, grades would probably not improve. That in turn could confirm Oliver's suspicion that I also was not on top of things, psychiatry and therapy was for the birds, an attitude I encountered regularly among smart, powerful but psychologically unsophisticated parents. I walked a tightrope. I had constant doubts as to whether I should continue, but thinking about it, 2 years into treatment Henry's academic slide had stopped. He had a B average, and he even began studying for the SATs. So, was I helping after all? Or just colluding?

In Henry's senior year, he moved in with his father in Tiburon after Charlette announced that she was moving back to Louisiana. This time, I insisted on a family session. Mother came in, dressed ready for a film shoot of "Gone with the Wind."

"I must confess, doctor, it's mostly for me, my career, I owe that to myself. I have sacrificed myself for these children all my life. And what do I get? Oliver is still messing around with the child support. Henry needs a man in his life. Don't you agree, Henry?" Charlette anticipated a "Bohemian" lifestyle, in which there was very little room for adolescent boys. Charlette patted Henry's hand with a smile.

As his mother's hand made contact, I could see a familiar posture: Henry went onto the watchtower, his face smooth and expressionless. He left his hand on the armrest, but there was no turning to mother, no meeting her gaze or taking her hand. Of course, Henry agreed with his mother. "Yeah, that's fine. I am spending so much time with dad, I might as well live there".

Because of his superior SAT scores and final grades, Henry was accepted at UC Santa Barbara. I saw Henry occasionally. He had a small group of friends at college, mostly from his sailing in Tiburon. He continued to struggle with grades, but he continually fended off any attempt of mine to link that to how his parents treated him. I was encouraged, however, because he started talking about his problems with women. His explanation of why his relationships were invariably tortured, lacking growth was that, "I guess I must be boring."

I found it difficult to take these statements seriously. Stiff and on guard, I could believe that his dates would complain about it. In describing his interactions with his girlfriends, he reported respect, fairness, kindness, and politeness. By his report, Henry treated women carefully, as if handling fragile, precious pieces of glass sculpture. I observed that with our female staff, he seemed relaxed and generous with his time. They always looked forward to his appointments, because he invariably would ask them politely about their lives, remember their names, and bring little gifts, such as chocolates and cards.

I asked him about how he started relationships. He reported a deep curiosity about his girlfriends' families asking many earnest questions about their upbringing. I often wondered where this came from, given what I knew about his family, but I was glad of it. However, underneath the courteous treatment of his dates, I sensed a carefully titrated distance, not too dissimilar from how he acted with me. In both therapy and dates, Henry was the one that controlled closeness and intimacy.

As he secured new dates after breakups and showed no interest in digging deeper into the issue, I was relegated to my familiar role: providing a psychotherapeutic cheering section on his search for a life's mate. Offers to explore dating more deeply were met by his dutifully making follow-up appointments, which he did not keep, citing various time pressures. I began to understand why Oliver reacted so angrily to Henry's failures: I, too, felt put aside, ignored, neutralized. But it was a restless neutrality: I often felt like I was walking on an English moor, where the ground could give way at any time.

And here it was: a letter from his mother with a death threat. I had just stepped into a bog. I was speechless. This is how he must feel at this moment. As I had time to catch my breath, I felt fear, then anger, almost immediately followed by worry. Fear, because of the open threat of the first line, anger, because how could Charlette do this to Henry; worry, because it was not immediately clear to me what the next steps were.

I repeated, "Where is she?"

Silence. Then a very shaky voice said, "I think she's in New Orleans, in her house. I probably should go there."

"Who can you call right now? Did you call the police?" I asked.

"No, I didn't. This may be just one of her stunts. She always pulls this crap, and then it turns out she was drunk and slept with one of her friends."

"Can you at least call her neighbors and some of these friends? And make immediate arrangements to go down there?" I asked. While that seemed initially to me the wrong move, perpetuating his old role as mother's guardian, once again "cleaning up Charlette's shit," it did seem the logical next step. But suddenly Henry wavered.

"I have to finish a bunch of stuff here, otherwise I flunk another semester. And then dad will have a major cow and threaten to withdraw all support—again. Plus, it's going to cost an arm and a leg to go down there on such short notice," he explained.

Here was his deep ambivalence about his mother. I said I would write a letter to make this a medical emergency, so he should not worry about cost. I rued the day that I did not force Charlette to be more involved in Henry's treatment. Could she be really playing these kinds of tricks? Was I overreacting?

"It seems I am more worried than you are," I observed.

A brief silence, then he murmured a breathy, "You don't know the half of it." More silence. Then he said with some resolve in his voice: "Ok, I stick to the plan and go down there."

He must have landed the next day in New Orleans, but there were no messages or phone calls, only my attempts to reach him. I oscillated between worry and fury. After 10 days, the front desk passed on a message that Henry was staying for his mother's funeral.

When Henry returned, it was spring break in Santa Barbara. He wanted a series of sessions before he returned. I put him on my schedule, half-expecting him not to show up. He came, even was early for his session. As Henry leaned back in his usual chair, I looked for signs of emotion. He began the session with a series of polite questions about how I had been, what kept me busy, and whether I had any plans for travel or sabbatical in the near future. I felt myself getting increasingly impatient and tense and finally stopped him.

"Henry, what happened to your mom?" I asked.

He threw his head back and closed his eyes and said, "That funeral was a joke. Bizarre, if you ask me."

"What happened?" I asked. "Last I heard from you, you were calling people and going to Louisiana."

"Oh, I didn't tell you? She committed suicide. Just like her brother. She used the same gun," he said flatly.

I had a hard time containing myself. Here was one of Henry's defenses he used to minimize his pain, avoid emotions, and keep the impression alive that he was working with me, while keeping me mostly in the dark. I had to remember what this defense accomplished for him, as it helped him get through the worst. As always, it took me a while to regain my composure. The net effect on me was that I only could manage a feeble Hallmark response.

"Oh, Henry, how horrible. I cannot imagine how that must feel," I said. All his emotion was in my voice. Henry remained composed, looked almost relieved.

I remembered dimly that the father and Henry had mentioned Beauregard's suicide in the first sessions. Father thought I ought to know because "there could be something genetic going on here", a view that Henry also wondered about. Charlette never confirmed or disconfirmed it. Her family never acknowledged it, and the reasons for his committing suicide were kept under close wraps.

As he followed up with details of Charlette's death, Henry's voice remained measured, punctuated by occasional expressions of disgust. I kept looking for sadness, grief, tears, trembling lips, but I saw none. After our phone call, he had taken a red eye without calling ahead to the police. He did try and reach some neighbors from the airport, but to no avail. He took a taxi through the sleeping Garden District. As he rode up to Charlette's house, he saw a large candelabra burning in the entry hall; otherwise, the house was dark and completely still. He went upstairs to his mother's bedroom. The door was open.

"There she was, Dr. Steiner. She lay on her bed, dressed in all black, her brother's shotgun resting across her chest. My first thought was: why is she sleeping with her brother's gun? Then I noticed the pool of blood on the sheets and the floor. I saw the hole in her chest. This was the way her brother killed himself. This was the same weapon Beauregard used," Henry said, and took a deep breath. I noticed a featherlike quiver in his jaw.

"How did you feel?" I asked. It took all I had to just say that. I really wanted to scream.

Henry leaned back in his armchair, looked up at the ceiling. His face was frozen, his eyes wide open, not a tear visible.

"On the flight down, I thought about what I was going to find. I didn't think she would do it. And not this way," he said. "But apparently it was the only thing left for her to do."

Henry could not elaborate on what he meant. He rubbed his eyes.

Suddenly, he shifted into a detailed account of his mother's funeral. I struggled: should I follow up on the desperate statement before? But then I thought this switch might help him get to his grief. I continued to listen. Charlette was buried at LaFayette Cemetery, not too far from the mansion she grew up in and where she had returned just a few years before. The funeral party assembled at the gravesite of the family, where her mother, father, and brother lay buried in their stone house, above ground. The small party stood by the tomb, waiting for the pallbearers to slide the casket into the grave's opening. Henry recognized almost all of the people who had come, except one couple. When he craned his neck, he could read their name on their wreath: John and Mary Proulx. Charlette had never spoken of them. The longer Henry spoke, the more furious he sounded, not sad.

"Ridiculous: Dad was there and his brother, Dick. Can you imagine? And one of the therapists from where she used to go to get dried out. Nobody from her side of the family. Some of the people from the galleries where she had shows – all men. That was it. And me and my sister." Henry said as his eyes turned to slits, and his left upper lip bared his teeth. He looked as if he had bitten into a rotten apple.

"Henry, you look disgusted. Why?" I asked.

"My Dad's brother! Dick! I told you about what happened at Christmas, when I was about 7, and my Dad was in the hospital having his appendix out. Dick came to stay with us to help. And when I got up Christmas morning, because I couldn't wait any longer, there was nothing under the tree. I went back to bed, but at six I could not stand it any longer and I knocked on mom's door. She came out in her skimpy night gown, and I see Dick in her bed. He was screwing his brother's wife while Dad was in the hospital!" he said.

Here it was again, the drawbridge going up, while Henry waved from the watchtower. But this time it did not work. He wiped his forehead vigorously with his hand, as if to erase the memory. His face contorted with pain. "I hop on my bike and go down to Mills Hospital where Dad was. I told him all about it. He was all doped up, after his operation. I was not sure he really got what I was saying. When I got home, mom skewers me in the hall: 'Where were you?' I tell her, then she yells at me: 'You broke the code! Men don't tell on men!' I had no idea what she was talking about. Then she said, 'Because of that, no Christmas'."

After Henry left, I still felt all his rage, impotence, disappointment, and disgust, like a garbage container for his unconscious. I began to understand what confused him when he received the letter: Charlette's suicide could be a solution for him in the short run. I was left with the uneasy feeling that part of the story was still missing. Henry had left the last session in a big hurry, his usual way to regain composure.

We had scheduled four more sessions after his return. He came for one, then went back to school, citing academic pressures. In this last session, he brought up more details of what life with mother had been like. She was drinking daily before, and after the divorce, many times a week to the point of complete drunkenness, unable to walk, vomiting, and losing control of her bladder and bowels. He and his sister would clean her up, return her to bed.

While drunk, she would attack children and Oliver mercilessly. Sometimes she would remember these episodes, mostly not. As I thought back to the beginning of therapy, I saw that I really did not grasp the seriousness of the situation at the time. Oliver habitually downplayed problems of living with mom; Charlette was entitled and oblivious at the same time. The entire family dynamic worked to keep the status quo. Neither Henry nor his sister ever told anyone. They did not want to get placed in foster care or with their father, which meant much scrutiny, control, and interference. When they approached Oliver, he brushed it off: "Your mother is an artist, she lives an artist's life. It was too much for me, but I am sure she is good for you." Both children became very good at disguising their home life, forgetting about it. They had to.

"Henry, I am beginning to understand better why it is so very difficult to grieve for your mother. You must be so enraged with her and Dad" I said.

"Not Dad. He didn't know anything about this," Henry replied.

"It is hard for me to believe that." I looked as gently at him as I could muster. What came was another bomb. He could not contain his rage, veins standing out on his neck.

"No, really," Henry said. "And as far as my mother goes, you have to remember that she was raped and molested for years by her brother. Her parents never did anything about that, because her father was a colonel and an upstanding citizen, and stuff like this did not go on in his family." Henry's furious release did not last long.

Once again, I was speechless and felt bound and paralyzed. I needed time to think and recover. But I could plant a seed. I noticed that time was almost up, so I said, "Henry, we have to start working on this. I know you are trying to bury it, but I am worried that it will come back to haunt you."

"Dr. Steiner, in all these years living with my family, I have gotten really good at making it all go away. It's only at times like this that it comes back. I am sure it will be gone again soon. I know it's your job to get to the bottom of this stuff, but what if I can live without doing that? Who says we have to do that? Therapists always want to stretch things out, don't they?" Henry said and looked at me with a challenge in his eyes. He left the economic implications of his statement hanging in the air.

"Henry, now you sound a little bit like your father. Here is what I think: I am all for letting sleeping dogs lie. But what if they dream? What if they wake up and bite?" I asked.

Henry nodded, "Fair enough. I'll think about this one".

Henry returned to campus and disappeared from my radar. I guess that was his answer. Maybe he had a point. Sometimes people live through hell, push it away, bury it, make up a whole other life in their minds and another identity, and then go on with their lives. Maybe Henry was one such person. I told myself he needed the time to heal again, and he had to pursue his studies. But I had mixed feelings. I let him know that I would be ready to see him again as soon as his schedule allowed. I did not think he was done with this topic. I believed that, sooner or later, Charlette would return, although I was not sure in what form or disguise.

It only took 2 months. Following his most recent breakup with another student, Henry began having nightmares.

"It's really weird. I am having this same dream I haven't had in years. I'm ten years old, and I am in the house in San Carlos. I wake up in the middle of the night because I hear something outside my room. I get the feeling there's someone out there. I get out of bed, open the door, look down the hall – and then I wake up, drenched in sweat," he said, looking like a terrified little boy.

This seemed like a repressed memory returning. He reported the identical elements of the dream, pushing them a bit further each time he described them. He looked completely anguished like I had never seen him before, sweating and wringing his hands. The details of the case emerging in the wake of his mother's suicide also fit: trauma after trauma, a drunken woman out of control, a distant and only superficially involved father, a boy who resembled father, and the proxy target for this mother's rage all provided the fitting context.

I could not be certain, however. I had to avoid leading him at all costs. I said, "You are describing the symptoms of a traumatic nightmare. Keep track of the dreams as they progress. It's scary, but let's keep working with it." I encouraged him to keep a notepad by his bedside, ready to write as soon as he woke up from the dream. Two sessions later, he began to see a figure in the hall, a dark shape, with something light around it. But before he could see more, he again awoke, his heart pounding. He began describing another feeling, but was unsure what to label it: fear, shame, something like that.

"I saw her," he said. "She was against a window. It's a woman, definitely a woman."

"Do you recognize her?" I began to feel afraid of what was about to come—anticipating Henry's reaction.

He looked blank, and it took him several minutes to answer. "Not sure, not sure." By now, his feeling ashamed had gotten really strong. "As if I'd done something wrong," he said as he blushed. Henry had to go through this hell mostly alone. Only after there was more clarity could I reach in and help. It was hard to see him leave after each session, as his etched memories emerged, one frame at a time, interrupted by overwhelming terror.

All of a sudden, there it was. "The figure comes out of my mom's bedroom – I wake up, frozen with fright, almost paralyzed. It's my mom,—just in her nighty. She wet herself again. She keeps bouncing off the wall, trying to steady herself with her hands. She keeps coming closer, comes towards me stumbling, says, 'Henry, you come here.' She's drunk again, she's hammered. She pushes me down to the floor, then rapes me," he said.

I felt as paralyzed as Henry, unable to say anything. The stupid thought ran through my mind: "I was right, I was right!", as if that mattered. I too am not immune to intellectualization. Finally, I managed this: "You must have been so terrified. And no one there to help."

Henry sat motionless, staring at his feet. "But Dr. Steiner, do you really think this happened? I could just be making it all up." He stared at me coldly, ready to pull the drawbridge up.

"I know it is very hard to cope with all this," I said. "But please take it seriously. The detail of the dream tells me it is etched, fits with your experience with your drunken mom that you have described. I am sure your sister also can help with this. She must have witnessed some of this."

Henry just sat there. Finally, he said, "You know, mother used to laugh, then say, 'With this little pecker, you'll never make a woman happy.' That really got me. I wanted to kill her when she said that."

Henry began to remember more and more of his early adolescent years. He and his sister compared notes. She confirmed much of what he remembered. The mixture of dread, shame, and excitement that awoke him in the night, the disgust which overwhelmed him.

As taxing as Henry's remembering was, it allowed me to make links to his problems with women. "No wonder you are so confused. All these contradictory feelings swirling around in you, uncontrolled, not put to rest. No wonder that your strongest reaction to your mother's death was disgust and disdain. I thought that you used that to defend against your grief, but I can see how your wanting revenge might have gotten the better of you."

Henry looked exhausted. "The whole thing in New Orleans was unreal," he said. "Like a soap opera."

"Very often when we go through extreme trauma, like you have, we step out of reality," I explained. "It becomes distant—we are just bystanders, watching ourselves on a stage."

Henry protested. "Ok, but why was it so bad? She never beat me, as drunk as she could get."

"Henry, trauma comes in many forms. Look, 10-year-old boys are not supposed to be the husbands or nurses of their drunkard mother. And all of these feelings going in you when you and your girlfriends become close: disgust, dread, shame, guilt. No wonder you struggle with intimacy as soon as you get close to women. How could you not?" I asked.

Henry just nodded. I was not sure he listened. "I know you are trying to help me. But it must have something to do with me."

As much as I wanted Henry to work through his trauma, it was just simply not possible for him to do so then. He cancelled the next session. The dreams had stopped. He needed to get back to Santa Barbara, everyday life, familiar territory. I wrote my last progress note very slowly. I ended it with: "She will be back. And I hope he will too." This much uncertainty, so much of a life in the balance, yet not in my office, not under control, is a psychiatrist's nightmare. But seeing Henry's frightened agony, his twisted face, years after all this happened, witnessing his painful search for a partner, I was ready for the next step. And I knew Oliver was wrong: Henry was a tough young man, I could help; he had lots of strength. But I had to be patient; it had to be under his control, not mine.

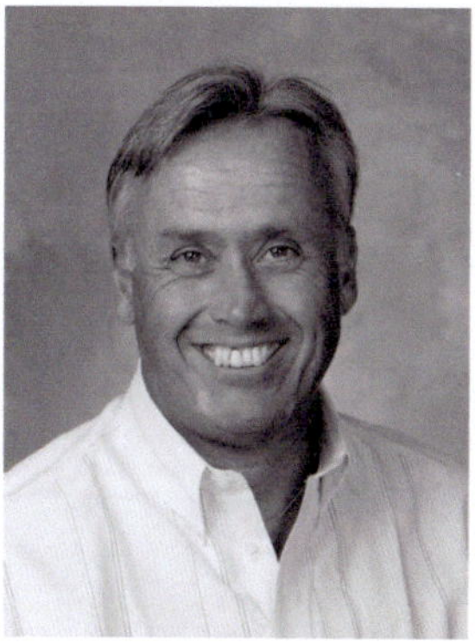

Dr. Hans Steiner (1946-2022) was a beloved and highly accomplished Professor Emeritus in the Department of Psychiatry & Behavioral Sciences of the Stanford University School of Medicine. He founded the Pegasus Physicians at Stanford. He authored and edited more than 500 articles, abstracts, reviews, and books. A nine time winner of the Outstanding Mentor Award from the American Academy of Child and Adolescent Psychiatry, he mentored Dr. Lisa Jacobs along with countless others. Dr. Jacobs and Dr. Steiner worked together on this anthology from 2019 until his death in 2022. Has served as the corresponding author on Dr. Steiner's story in an effort to preserve his work and his last literary contribution.

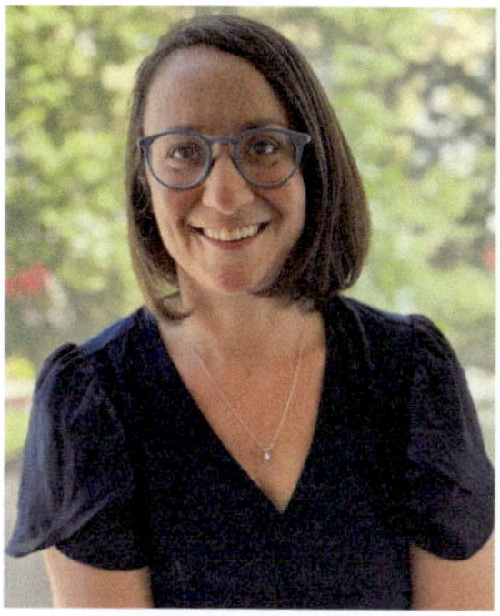

Dr. Lisa Jacobs is a child, adolescent, and adult psychiatrist in private practice in New York City and New Jersey. She serves as an Adjunct Clinical Assistant Professor in the Department of Psychiatry & Behavioral Sciences of the Stanford University School of Medicine. She serves as a group leader in The Pegasus Physician Writers at Stanford. She graduated from Cornell University and completed her medical training at Brown University, The University of Pennsylvania, and Stanford University. She is the 2019 winner in the prose category of the Irvin D. Yalom Literary Award for her short story, "Trapped in a Blizzard with a Politician in Withdrawal."

12 Six Feet Apart

Richard Wu

This is why we are here: because we want to help people. Because we enjoy solving problems. Because we are fascinated by human anatomy, or love hearing patients' stories, or have watched too many episodes of *Scrubs*. Some of us were inspired early on by a doctor or nurse in the family. Others started out elsewhere—*I was a software engineer at Microsoft, I taught middle school music classes, I was a professional swimmer and almost made it to the Olympics*—before we changed course to study medicine.

We have come from near and far. Some of us are natives of the windswept Texas prairies, where we have grown accustomed to sudden tornado warnings in the summer and bombardments of hail (but almost never snow) in the winter. Some of us have come from up north, from New York or New Jersey or Illinois, where we never had to crank up the air conditioning before and have grown bored of seeing snow year after year. Others have come from even further away, like India and Korea, fighting off jet lag during the first few days of our virtual medical school orientation on Zoom.

We are wide-eyed and hopeful from the start, even as we hear the words, *COVID-19 safety precautions* and *virtual classes*, and *no cadaver dissections this year*, and *in-person simulation activi-*

R. Wu (✉)
Psychiatry and Behavioral Sciences, Johns Hopkins Hospital, Baltimore, MD, USA

J. Pien et al. (eds.), *Onward*,
https://doi.org/10.1007/978-3-032-15776-8_12

ties once a week. We move into our new apartments while wearing hand-sewn face masks, or disposable surgical masks, or even N95 respirators if we can get ahold of them. We try not to worry about how much longer this pandemic might keep dragging along, or how many of us might be infected in the upcoming semester. As we lug mattresses and chairs and suitcases into our new rooms, our steps feel both light and heavy at the same time.

***

The first semester of medical school unfurls ahead, and we settle into the routine of virtual classes: 15 biology lectures, 5 anatomy lectures, 1 embryology lecture, and 1 histology lecture per week. We attend classes while wearing pajamas at our beds or living room couches, without our hair or makeup done. Sometimes we show up to Zoom sessions with our pet dog or cat in our lap. We watch video lectures whenever we decide to be awake: at 9:00 AM in the morning, or 2:00 PM in the afternoon, or 3:00 AM in the middle of the night.

As we study, our caffeine consumption is matched only by our consumption of biomedical alphabet soup. *Staphylococcus aureus. Vestibulocochlear nerve. Sphingomyelin. Inferior mesenteric artery. Ganciclovir*. In one video lecture, we watch our professor cut apart a human cadaver's arm and shoulder to show us how to navigate the brachial plexus and its tangled web of neuronal spaghetti. In another lecture, our professor slices open a cadaver's skull to extract the brain, and as we hear about the cerebrum and cerebellum and brainstem, our eyes are momentarily lost within that brain's labyrinth of swirling folds.

Once a week, we don masks and face shields for our in-person classroom simulation activities. We practice partial physical examinations on each other in groups of three or four, our hearts racing and our hands a bit unsteady as we fumble our way through taking blood pressure measurements, listening to heart pulses, looking inside ears with an otoscope. *Practice makes perfect*, we tell ourselves in muffled voices, and as we listen to the *lub-dub, lub-dub* of someone else's heart thumping through our stethoscopes, our nervous smiles are hidden away beneath our layered masks and face shields.

***

Over Zoom lectures, our medical school professors teach us about the COVID-19 virus. We learn about ACE2 receptors and spike proteins, and the D614G mutation. We chart out constellations of symptoms—coughing, chills, fever, fatigue, nausea, vomiting, diarrhea, loss of taste or smell—which sometimes may present with all of the above, or some of the above, or none of the above. We hear again and again about airborne transmission, about social distancing and wearing masks, about washing hands with soap and water.

But our medical school professors don't teach us anything about what to do when our grandmother, our aunt and uncle, our family friend tests positive for COVID-19. They don't teach us what to say when our family phones us to ask, *What should we do? You're almost a doctor, right?* They don't teach us how to deal with the feeling of being caught between heartbeats, of being suspended breath by breath, unable to do anything but wait.

***

We pick up our white coats shortly before Halloween. *Nice costume*, we joke to ourselves, *you actually look like a doctor.*

And then we remark, *This is the cleanest that our white coats will ever be.*

Soon afterward, we begin to practice physical examinations on actors who pretend to be our patients. Each of us learns the drill: line up in the simulation center hallway under the glowing fluorescent lights, march down the stairs, find the assigned individual room number. Knock at the door. Enter the imitation-doctor's office, where a gowned actor-patient waits on a hospital bed. Sanitize hands, put on gloves, pretend to be a doctor. *Hi, I'm here to do a physical exam, is now a good time?* we say to our actor-patient, before stammering, *First…do you mind…lowering your gown?* Our faces redden as we force those words out through our face masks, to people who are old enough to be our own parents or grandparents.

Look like a doctor. Pretend to be a doctor. Even if we don't feel like doctors yet, we tell ourselves again and again, *Fake it until you make it.*

***

Outside our apartments, a chill seeps into the air. Our grandmother and our family friend pass away from COVID-19. Our aunt and uncle survive.

The medical school professors do not teach us how to mourn and study at the same time, how to keep ourselves from drowning with one foot dragged down by loss, and the other foot sinking under a tidal wave of schoolwork. And they do not teach the rest of us that there are an uncountable number of ways to say, *I'm so sorry for your loss*, all of them numbingly inadequate.

This is when we first notice a sense of burnout creeping up on us. We fail our first class, right after that time when we were busy consoling two friends who were grieving deaths in their own families. We are dumped by our college boyfriend of four years, and in the following days, our sobs shatter the glassy silence of our one-person apartment. We check our phone during a study break, only to see a message saying that an old friend from high school is dead, rumored to be from suicide. The national news topics don't bring much comfort, either: a looming election, the COVID-19 pandemic, systemic racism, angry wildfires blazing out of control across California.

We speed through video lecture after video lecture in the quarantined spaces of our apartment rooms. But even though our heads are overstuffed with medical terminology and drug lists and countless mnemonics, our hearts feel a bit gaping and empty.

***

We watch video recordings of our practice physical examinations. We watch ourselves step into the imitation-doctor's-office, complete with our white coats. Looking like doctors. Pretending to be doctors. Our recorded selves say nervously *Hi, I'm here to do a physical exam, is now a good time?*

We watch ourselves start the physical examination without first putting on gloves. We watch ourselves forget to disinfect the stethoscope, or hit the wrong part of the actor-patient's knee with a reflex hammer, or accidentally skip over that one step where we were supposed to palpate for lymph nodes. Our recorded voices sound a little too fast or high-pitched, and our white coats look a little too white.

As we count one mistake after another, our throats tighten and our hands grow sweaty. We find ourselves wondering whether we will ever feel like real doctors, or whether we will always just be pretending like this, red-faced and stammering, our flashy white coats nothing more than make-believe doctor costumes.

***

We start to unload the words, *Zoom fatigue* and *stressed out* and *so unbelievably alone* and *everyone is struggling*. When was the last time we saw our family? *My family's in Korea, and I haven't seen them in almost a year.* How much longer will we have to live like hermits? *I'd gladly take a B on our next final if I could have a normal social interaction in the next seven months.* Is there anything that our medical school administration can do? *They say that they hear us and they're sorry, but they seem to get defensive every time we try to give feedback, and sometimes I almost feel like they don't really care about us.*

At times, we regress back to our childhoods and play Minecraft or Super Smash Bros for five hours straight. We starve ourselves and then gorge on cookies-and-cream ice cream, gummy worms, sour-cream-and-onion potato chips, spicy instant ramen. We start fostering a cat in our apartment, hoping that the socially-distanced landlord will never walk in or take notice of our new guest.

***

As the weather grows colder and the semester drags on, we continue to practice physical examinations. We've begun to look and sound nearly half-mechanical—but at least we're no longer stammering or blushing—when we ask our actor-patients to disrobe. We make sure to put on gloves, to disinfect our stethoscope, to palpate for lymph nodes in the right places.

In our video lectures, our professors teach us about parasitic worms: *Loa loa* squirming inside an eyeball, *Ascaris lumbricoides* wriggling out of a child's nose. Did we know how people used to treat *Ascaris* roundworms before medications became available? *You would starve the patient for a few days. The patient would go to sleep. You'd wave a piece of warm bacon in front of their nose. And then the hungry roundworms would smell the bacon and wriggle out through the patient's nostrils.*

We wonder if this could be the treatment for medical student burnout too: go to sleep (medical students are usually already half-starved and sleep-deprived), put a piece of warm bacon in front of our noses, wait for that visceral sense of burnout to come wriggling out through our nostrils like a writhing swarm of hungry, hungry worms.

***

When we are feeling alone and need a hug, we put on face masks and meet up outside, standing six feet apart from one another. We face each other and spread our arms wide into a distance-hug and embrace the open air, giggling self-consciously. Rays of sunlight tickle our foreheads from above, and we stand there with our arms stretched out like the horizon, suspended right between the earth and sky.

While our professors lecture us on the differences between cholinergic neurons and adrenergic neurons, we put together care packages for our classmates who have lost family members to COVID-19. We make and illustrate cards, add some succulent plants, stick in some extra energy drinks or granola snacks or chocolate bars. We write notes of encouragement to our classmates, bake each other cookies, reach out to ask, *Are you doing okay?*

We try not to forget why we are here: because we want to help people.

***

The announcement that we've been waiting for lands into our lives near the end of our first semester. We find out while packing our bags for the Thanksgiving holiday, or while babysitting our cousin's toddlers, or right after volunteering to call the geriatric clinic's patients. Our heart is hammering in our chest as we sit still for a moment, our eyes gazing upward and our chin tilted back, and we let out a breath before saying, *Finally*.

We think of our grandmother, our family friend who never got to see this day. We think back to our virtual medical school orientation four months ago, when we still had no idea what medical school in a pandemic would look like. We think back to the first time we sewed a face mask ten months ago, when we had hoped that COVID-19 would be under control by the start of medical school.

We know that we won't be the first to receive the new vaccine; that honor goes to the frontline workers who are treating COVID-19 patients. But when we hear that we might be vaccinated at the start of the next semester, we tell ourselves, *Hang in there, everything will be okay.*

***

It's the last day of the semester, right after our final exam. We're standing outside our apartments in the crisp (but snowless) December afternoon, with our noses and mouths warmed up by the heat trapped in our face masks. The wind rustles through a nearby tree's yellowing leaves, and the sun shines down from overhead.

We stand together in a circle—six feet apart from one another—and we spread our arms out wide. We smile and giggle under our masks as we distance-hug for the last time of this semester, with our arms embracing the air, with our hearts embracing one another.

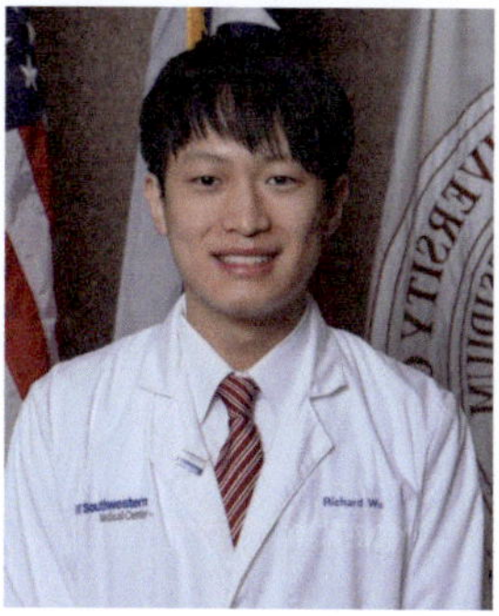

Richard Wu is a current psychiatry resident physician at the Johns Hopkins Hospital and obtained his medical degree from the University of Texas Southwestern Medical School. He is passionate about the intersection between medicine and the arts and enjoys writing stories, creating art, and composing music. Richard was recognized with an Honorable Mention for the 2021 Irvin David Yalom Literary Award and an Honorable Mention in the 2020 Paul Kalanithi Writing Contest. His writing has been featured in *Bellevue Literary Review*, *The Healing Muse*, *Lifelines*, *Family Medicine*, *Nature*, and other publications.

Portraits of a Mr. E

13

Steve Asch

Dr. David Hopper sat down on Mr. E's empty hospital bed. It felt good to rest on the blank white sheets for just a minute. Hiding behind the bed curtain, he let his tired eyes close. The wartime sounds of the History Channel fought with beeping I.V. poles and heart monitors.

"Where is Mr. E?" he wondered, opening his eyes.

Mr. E was the last patient on his morning rounds of the neuro-rehabilitation ward. A bearded man's photo stared back at him, taped to the wall above the bedside. Blue eyes, red hair, he hugged a smiling young woman turned three quarters away from the camera.

"Mr. E?" he guessed and glanced at his watch.

He flicked off the TV and caught a reflected glimpse of his grey hair and white coat in the crackling dark screen. Families often posted photos to create a familiar and friendly environment for disoriented patients. The pictures were also supposed to humanize the often uncommunicative patients to the staff. Dr. Hopper paid those pictures little notice. Old vacation snapshots

First published in the Pegasus Review

S. Asch (✉)
Department of Medicine, Stanford University School of Medicine,
Palo Alto, CA, USA

J. Pien et al. (eds.), *Onward*,
https://doi.org/10.1007/978-3-032-15776-8_13

predominated, healthy long-ago avatars of his stroke victims and their consorts on the beach, like an antique Facebook feed.

This wall was different. Many more pictures decorated it than usual, some overlapping. Some belonged to the usual family photo album genre, like the first one he had noticed, but others did not. The presumptive Mr. E appeared in a couple in the middle, but the surrounding pictures mostly had no people in them at all. "Is that an abstract painting or a photograph?" Dr. Hopper asked himself. He scooted to the head of the bed to get a closer look at what appeared to be an aerial view of a crimson river delta. It reminded him of a pathology tissue slide from medical school.

"He is in the scanner at the moment," a woman's voice said from out of view. Dr. Hopper jumped up from the bed and turned in the direction of the voice, feeling like he was somehow trespassing. A thin, elegant fiftyish woman in a scarf stood in the doorway.

"Oh, okay. I'm Dr. Hopper," he replied. "The neurologist." He extended his hand. She shook it crisply, brushing the curtain with her elbow.

"Hello. Very nice to meet you. Helen," she said. He wondered if she was the smiling woman in the picture of the couple at the party. It was hard to tell.

"Nice to meet you too. Uh, are you…"

"Yes. I'm his wife." Was that a British accent? He pressed his lips together into a smile facsimile. He could not do a proper consult without the patient, but maybe he could get a head start by talking to the wife now and examining Mr. E later.

"Good. I was hoping you could tell me a few things about your husband. Would that be okay?" She nodded. "Why don't you start by telling me how your husband got here." Mrs. E arched her eyebrows.

"You know, I just told this story to that young doctor. Perhaps you two should talk." She actually sniffed.

"Yes, I understand," he sighed. "Still, it's best that I hear the original version for myself."

She obliged him. Dr. Hopper took a blank index card from the stack in his pocket. On it, he wrote a capital E and the last four digits of the medical record number at the top, the minimum identifying information needed to access the patient's electronic medical record, and he let Helen take the lead. As he wrote, she meandered her way down the descending path that her husband's health had taken over the past years and weeks. For someone that did not want to tell the story again, she certainly took her time doing it. When she stopped, Dr. Hopper took inventory of what they had discussed.

E1962
71 yr old male. Past medical history: Stage IV Gleason 8 prostate CA s/p radiation for bone mets, androgen deprivation. History of present illness: Sudden dense expressive and receptive aphasia, R sided weakness. CT: moderate L sided infarct, mostly confined to language areas. No neuro improvement post 2 wks of Rx. Course complicated by aspiration pneumonia. Abnl swallowing study. Feeding tube placed. I.V. fluids @40cc/hr, antibiotics. Transferred for rehab.

He put the card back in his pocket, thanked Mrs. E, and turned to leave.

"Did you like the picture?" she asked.

"Sorry?" he said with his hand on the door.

"The picture you were gazing at so intently." Her extended first finger swung toward it like she was conducting an orchestra. "The crimson one."

He followed her finger. "Oh yes. Very nice." Dr. Hopper left.

When he came back, she was gone, replaced by Mr. E. lying sideways in his bed. His eyes were still blue, but his hair was white. A plastic feeding tube dangled from his nose. A crust of dried saliva and skin caked the corners of his mouth. He was breathing loudly.

Dr. Hopper leaned in close. "Hi, I'm Dr. Hopper!" He always talked loudly when meeting patients for the first time as they were often hard of hearing. Mr. E's eyes shifted toward him for a second. "I'm going to examine you now, okay?" He took out his reflex hammer. Mr. E shifted in his bed and blinked.

Later, Dr. Hopper pulled out his index cards and placed them on his cubicle desk. He logged on to Epic, the hospital's electronic medical record system. The software's corporate logo came up along with its eyerollingly grandiose tag line: "Like the Iliad or Odyssey, our electronic health records chronicle the story of a patient's health over time." David Hopper's weary mind wandered: his father, the late Dr. Jesse Hopper, was an epic storyteller. David's father would regale his family at the dinner table with stories from work, like the time he met a man with three nipples. The elder Dr. Hopper often employed his patients and knew their families, which David found awkward and embarrassing. When the aforementioned man arrived at the Hoppers' home to fix their water heater, David's father pointed to his own chest and whispered, "That's the guy!"

The younger Dr. Hopper did not take over the family practice or grow to rival his father's narrative powers. The intricacies of the brain fascinated him; the ghost in the machine did not. He loved sifting through the grey details of the neurologic exam and the scans to uncover the golden nugget of a diagnosis. His skill at extracting the essential meaning from a complex world evoked the admiration of his colleagues at Bay Area Neurology Group, but for different reasons. As the managing partner, he built risk-benefit spreadsheets that helped make them the most successful neurology practice in the West.

He pulled out the index card labeled E1962. He typed that into the computer, then clicked on Mr. E's name. He distilled the facts and sorted them into the predefined data fields: present illness, past illnesses, and so on.

The only narrative part was a short paragraph describing the assessment and therapeutic plan. Rehabilitation patients presented few of the intellectual challenges Dr. Hopper relished, and all of the interesting but, in retrospect, fruitless work had already been done during Mr. E's ICU stay. The scans showed the whole picture anyway: a dark blotch obscuring the speech center and much more. A pretty bleak picture. Dr. Hopper signed an order for physical therapy and wrote a few formulaic phrases about "monitoring neurologic progress," though he doubted there would be much improvement, especially in the presence of such an advanced cancer.

When he was done, he found a link to Mr. E's scanned advance directive from his oncologist, dated 11 months ago. It named Mrs. E as the surrogate decision maker. The box indicating I do not want life-prolonging treatment if I become unconscious and, to a reasonable degree of medical certainty, I will not regain consciousness was checked. In Sect. 2.3 ("Other Wishes"), a precise but flowing hand had written: No artificial breathing or feeding.

Dr. Hopper had trouble with advance directive forms. They used commonplace and medically imprecise language, making it difficult for him to accurately ascertain the intent. And how could the old Mr. E know what the present Mr. E would want, in any case? Dr. Hopper felt the forms often revealed grievous ignorance of the patient's future state and treatment options and thus warranted revision in the face of new clinical circumstances. Instead, surrogates (as family members are known in the vocabulary of such forms) and many doctors treated the forms like holy writs and anguished over their meaning. In this case, the objective evidence, the published clinical trials, did not speak clearly for or against artificial feeding. But the form did.

Come to think of it, why did Mr. E have a feeding tube when the form clearly said he didn't want one?

Once again, Dr. Hopper clicked through Epic to find the advance directive. He flitted down to the line about avoiding life-prolonging treatment. Check. Hmm.

He frowned, then narrowed his eyes. Inconsistencies and contradictions bothered him, and this was not a small one. There was a lot of debate about feeding tubes for stroke patients. It was not clear that they prolonged life even in patients with moderate-sized strokes like Mr. E. Patients' preferences mattered a lot. Talking to surrogates was far from his favorite task, but he reluctantly wrote on Mr. E's index card: Ask wife re feeding tube. Bring the AD form.

Portrait of a Lover

"You were always as talented a pickup artist as the other kind of artist," Helen Edgewater told her silent husband lying next to her in the hospital bed. The morning light from the window did his pallor no kindness.

She met Sean at the National Gallery in London. She was copying the seventeenth-century Rokeby Venus, that shameless hussy, for an art history module at University College. In it, a flitty Cupid holds a mirror to his nude mother. Venus lies on her side, vainly contemplating her reflection. When the Rokeby Venus was 265 years old, a suffragette slashed her scandalous canvas flesh in protest of the objectification of womankind, necessitating some artful surgery. Helen thought she looked none the worse for wear.

Helen was struggling to copy the dull and hazy reflection of Venus' face in Cupid's mirror. She was perched on the edge of a bench intently erasing pencil shading in her sketchbook when she felt someone looking over her shoulder.

"Better than the original, I think," Sean flattered her in a broad American voice. She instantly recognized his ginger hair and beard and piercing eyes from his publicity photo in the new Saatchi Gallery brochure.

Trying to overcome the dizzy feeling of nearness to fame, she quickly tried for the upper hand. "Shall I take that as a compliment or an insult from a minimalist?" she quipped.

She intended it as flirtatious banter, but, in retrospect, could he not have thought it absurdly snooty? He laughed anyway and sat down beside her, and they tossed witticisms at each other for a half hour. Then he got her phone number.

Helen fell in love, irretrievably, wholeheartedly, unconsciously, unintentionally, physically, mentally, nobody-could-talk-her-out--of-it in love. Oh, and Sean seemed "quite interested in her too," she explained to her friends. Her patrician parents thought the age difference a scandal, her classmates thought it a career-ending move, but a hop or two across the pond and Soho Helen Sinclair became San Francisco Helen Edgewater.

Helen felt a wave of nostalgia (and love, again) for the Sean of those heady and passionate days. The paint and brewing coffee smell of his Haight-Ashbury studio came back to her. A national glossy magazine ran a glam picture of them embracing at a posh gallery opening, next to a spread depicting his blue square series. Collectors competed to have him at dinner to show off his cleverness and his paintings, and she was his pretty and witty foil. She wasn't the only one who thought Sean's grand plans might come to pass.

They might have, but they didn't. The solo shows began featuring newer artists, and the dinner invitations petered out. Sean borrowed money to keep up appearances. He changed styles. "I think minimalism has long since reached its maximum," he wisecracked while theatrically stubbing out his ever-present cigarettes. Late middle age found him painting less and teaching at a university better known for engineering and medicine than art.

Helen felt distinctly unsuited for this new role of young faculty wife. Despite or perhaps because of their increasing emotional distance, she told Sean she wanted a family. Two sad miscarriages later, she felt that she was also distinctly unsuited for procreation. Sean halfheartedly suggested a surrogate mother, but Helen said no one was going to have her baby for her.

Instead, she began restoring paintings at the university's museum. It was a painstaking job, but Helen was brilliant at it. Sean said she had X-ray vision to see through the grime of centuries to the artist's vision. She actually did use the radiographic facilities at the medical school to examine the underpainting. Sometimes she saw abandoned figures, overpainted faces, even completely different paintings below their well-known surfaces. She relished those hidden layers of history and meaning. Many more choices went into restoration than most museumgoers realized, far beyond just removing the dirt. Did the artist know the subject's alabaster complexion would fade to cream a lifetime in the future? Perhaps he was painting for the ages, and Helen's brightening agents undermined that goal. Sean said no one really painted for the ages; they painted for the moment, or more likely for the money. Still, in her own small way, Helen felt she was adding her own story to the work, like the Chinese scholars who put their red ownership stamps on their paintings.

Sean also adapted and learned from his scientific colleagues. In another radical stylistic shift, he began a series of small, meticulously-painted-over human photomicrographs. Cigar-shaped muscle cells simplified with red and black, globular adipose tissue slices rendered a delicious yellow, and ovarian cancer biopsies boldly streaked grey and green, all populated his studio's easels. Sean told Helen and more than one skeptical art critic that he had invented a new kind of figurative painting, a new kind of interior landscape. He called them microportraits. Helen was half-certain he was half-joking, but she honestly admired the quirky bravado of the statement and the abstract expressionistic visual impact of the paintings. In any case, they did not exactly revive his flagging career.

Neither the sexual harassment accusation nor the threatened paternity suit was from a biology graduate student involved in the project. Oh, he seemed sorry, but the prospect that someone else might have had Sean's child was a deep wound that cut through their marriage. After a trial separation, they managed to paper it over. However, the repair was indeed paper-thin, and they withdrew into themselves to avoid testing it. Their playful verbal fencing retreated, and bitterness, sarcasm, and silence took its place.

Interrupting this long internal monologue, she cast her eyes on the back of Sean's head. "Do you even remember that awful girl's name? You know, dear, the one that gave us herpes?" Helen asked her mute and unresponsive husband. She willed herself to forget the woman's name, but did not succeed.

Thus, she remembered, their precious passion wilted away in more ways than one when Sean came home from the urologist with news. "He said Viagra might help us," a quivering smile peeking from beneath the grey beard. "But it won't help the prostate cancer."

But the prostate cancer had helped them, unexpectedly. It tapped a well of kindness under their polished surfaces and damaged connection that neither had heretofore easily seen in the other. She felt for his unmanning suffering and existential distress, and he felt for her fading future as a nursemaid and middle-aged widow. She helped him painfully mount the table where the enormous machine irradiated his cancer-riddled bones. He helped her clean the Bonnard portrait of the painter's wife, Marthe. After several months, they both took leaves of absence. They spent afternoons roaming museums and cataloguing his work. The emasculating medicine made his skin smooth and soft to the caress, and as he gradually lost weight, he regained some of his old gauntness. So compassion replaced passion, and some of their erstwhile playfulness returned.

Back in London to visit her parents, they sat again before the Rokeby Venus. Helen reclined on the bench, held out a compact mirror, and, aping the painting, applied some rouge.

"What would you do without me?" she vamped into the mirror. His sad eyes, magnified by his glasses, did not crinkle into amusement as she had hoped.

Instead, he asked her, "What will you do without me?"

She put the mirror down and sat up and looked at him directly. "Sean, really, the doctors said you could live for years."

"Maybe. What if I don't want to, though?"

"What do you mean?"

"I mean I already feel so diminished, you know, like damaged goods." He pointed to the back of Venus' neck, where she had been slashed. "I wonder if I've already done the important things by now."

"Of course not, you ninny. You can always paint me."

"That's the test then." He continued in an exaggerated Oxbridge accent. "If I cahn't paint you, I just cahn't go on." The mock melodrama hid something, she thought. He touched her face, pretending to adjust her makeup.

Back home 2 weeks later, she turned to him in bed and he did not answer to his name.

In the ambulance to St. Catherine Community Hospital, she found that she really was not ready to let him go, damaged goods or not. Sean had said no heroic measures, but why should it be up to just him? He had designated her to be his surrogate, but surrogacy was not all she wanted. For a change, Helen wanted to be the heroine, the protagonist, not just the interpreter. She was the one bearing the burden and she welcomed it. She would tend to him and to their lost future. She would continue to restore their love in her own way with whatever time they had left.

The next day, at the suggestion of the intensive care unit nurses, she brought some old pictures to help him remember who he was. She squeezed between the bed and the IV pole and sat next to her husband. First, she taped the pseudofamous magazine clipping of them embracing in the art gallery on the bedside wall where he might see it if he were lying on his side, which he often was since being admitted to the hospital.

"What do you think, Sean?" she asked. "That was a fine party, wasn't it?" She did not expect an answer, but perhaps the nurses were right, and the combination of the image of them together with the sound of her voice would help him. He did turn those baby blue eyes toward him, she thought, and the corners of his mouth rose a bit.

More pictures went up with careful effort over the next half hour or so. She surveyed her handiwork. Adjacent to the first picture, Sean and Helen squinted beside a Roman fountain into a sunrise after a long night out. Below that, they ate pastries in a forgotten cafe somewhere in England. To the left, he had snapped a shot of her looking up from a book at the beach, wrapped against the breeze. To the right, she had taken a picture of him laughing at an unseen joke, paintbrush in hand. Many of the nurses who wandered by paused to take in the "assemblage" as she had begun calling it to herself. As they put tubes in him or took waste out, some even remarked how handsome he had looked.

The day after that, she brought in the catalogue box of his signed microportraits. The doctors said he had lost too much weight, so she took out the fat cell microportrait and taped it in its yellow glory below yesterday's grouping. For good measure, she found a rhythmic brown one of the protuberant villi lining the small intestine and overlapped it a bit with the fat cells and the pastry picture. Then she tried to spoon-feed him the gooey food provided by the hospital, though he drooled most of it out. For strength, muscle cells looking like red spaceships in their own microportrait flew into the assemblage from the left, but fell short of landing on the beach picture. Spiculated, towering, bright white bone microportraits strengthened the bottom and warded off more painful spine metastases.

Of course, the stroke was the main event. Helen pulled out a fluorescent green neuron network on a black background and attached it to the top of the Roman fountain. She thought this might increase blood flow to the damaged brain tissue. "Come to think of it, maybe the red blood cell microportraits would help the flow too," she thought, so she taped up a portrait of two groups of red spheres next to the neurons for good measure.

The critics that regularly paraded through the hospital room gave her latest work mixed reviews. Mostly, people just filed by and either did not notice or glanced at them and said nothing. A priest (it was a Catholic hospital) said they looked very happy in the fountain picture. When people asked about the more abstract ones, she just said that Sean was an artist and that they were some of his latest paintings. She left it at that. The priest said he didn't care much for modern art but liked the colors, and he thought the assemblage as a whole had a kind of sacred feeling. "Of course, that happens to me a lot," the priest added. A phlebotomist said the blood cell microportraits looked like blood cells, so that was a bit encouraging. Not that she gave them much of a clue, but no one seemed to really catch on to her healing intent.

Maybe the problem was that she was not addressing the underlying condition, the cancer itself. That night at home, she searched the web for images of "prostate cancer Gleason score 8" on Sean's enormous high-definition monitor. The cells looked like estuarine islands viewed from the air. She tried drawing them unsatisfactorily on a sketch pad, which was not surprising as she had not really composed anything since leaving graduate school so long ago. Changing tactics, she printed out a color picture about the size of the other microportraits on heavy stock paper. She covered the islands carefully in crimson paint from Sean's studio, and painted the river portions a lighter red. She then searched for an image of healthy prostate tissue. It was much more uniform, so she just used the crimson paint for the repeating round parts and a light grey for the interstices. After a moment's hesitation, she signed Sean's name to both. The next morning, her prostate portraits joined the assemblage.

Sean's apparent awareness of his surroundings did not really improve over those days. Worse yet, he began to wheeze and gurgle, and Helen's heart sank. The doctors said that he had an infection in his lungs that was caused by choking on his own saliva. Helen added a light-filled lung microportrait from Sean's collection and a salivary gland of her own creation, putting them on opposite sides of the assemblage. The doctors pushed antibiotics through his IV and kept him on his side with his head up. They also told her to stop spoon-feeding him. His breathing seemed to improve.

After 10 days, Helen began to realize that Sean might never fully regain consciousness. The intensive care unit doctor asked her if she and Sean had ever talked about this eventuality. Of course they had, and not just that one time in the art museum. Feeling like she was cheating on an exam, she brought out the advance directive form from her portfolio. He had filled it out at the oncologist's office soon after the diagnosis and showed it to her. She was to take it with her if he were ever hospitalized and could not speak for himself. Three nights earlier, she took out the fine brushes she used for art restoration and carefully whited out the "Other Wishes" section where he had indicated that he did not want artificial breathing or feeding. With a fine pen, she changed the check box from not wanting life-prolonging treatment to wanting it and then adjusted the date to a more recent one. She showed this retouched form to the doctor, telling him that Sean was not ready to give up. Neither was she, and that day they placed the feeding tube in his nose.

Helen realized that, no matter how she felt, healing Sean was not the only or perhaps even the main purpose of her artwork. Maybe the priest had it right after all, and she should focus more on honoring Sean's life and their love. She brought in a reproduction of one of his minimalist blue squares, probably his most famous work. She put it next to the picture of him laughing with the paintbrush. It brought out the color in his eyes. She taped a picture of the Rokeby Venus, in all its evanescent fleshy radiance, next to the fountain photo. Lastly, she placed a photo of Bonnard's painting of his beloved dead wife, the one Helen restored, next to the Venus.

Then, for the first time since before the ambulance ride, she cried.

The day of the transfer, she brought in her large-format digital camera to document the assemblage. Then she meticulously deconstructed it, image by image, from newest to oldest, and placed them carefully back in her portfolio. She rushed to their new room to find a young assistant doctor from the neurorehabilitation team in her way, asking the same tiresome questions they all did. She answered the bare minimum and shooed him off. Then she reinstalled the assemblage in its new spot on the wall where Sean would soon be, oldest image to newest, intermittently comparing this second incarnation to the photos she had taken earlier in the day. She laid down where he would be to check the viewing angles and then went out to the nurses' station to ask them when Sean would arrive from the scanner.

When she returned, she was surprised to find Dr. Hopper sitting in their new bed examining the prostate portrait. It was their bed now, sort of, and she took silent offense.

He wanted to know the same history that his assistant, or whoever that was, had just taken from her. Annoyed that Sean would be gone for some time, she expanded her role in the sad story. She made sure to mention the herpes and to project an air of selfless doting, but carefully omitted any mention of the advance directive.

"Did you like the picture?" she asked afterwards. He gave a polite but blank reply, like most. Really, people could take more of an interest, she thought on the way home that night.

When Dr. Hopper came back the next day, he looked a bit agitated. He hovered at bedside, blocking her view of the assemblage.

"Mrs. Edgewater, this is not, ah, easy to discuss," he said after they had talked about the fluids and such, "but I wonder if you and Mr. Edgewater ever talked about, well, about his wishes?"

"Well yes, of course" she said. "His most fervent wish was that he had never contracted cancer of the prostate."

"Mrs. Edgewater, I think you know what I mean. Did the two of you ever discuss how he would want to be treated in a situation like this, when he was not able to communicate."

"Do you really think we should be talking about this here in front of him?" she asked. Sean, propped up with a pillow, stared at them. Dr. Hopper nodded and tilted his head toward the door.

Outside the room, he said, "I doubt he can understand us, Mrs. Edgewater."

"How can you know that?"

"I can't really. He is pretty debilitated from his cancer. Most of his brain is still fine, but his scans show a lot of damage to the areas of the brain that understand and produce speech. If we're honest, I'm not sure he will ever recover that ability."

Helen nodded and started to say that the old Sean would not want to live in the world Dr. Hopper described, his long and fading search for beauty derailed forever, his audience reduced to just her, his stage to a hospital bed. She stopped herself though. How could she be certain of that?

Dr. Hopper brought out the printed copy of the advance directive. "This is a form he filled out in the oncologist's office a year ago. It might help you. Maybe you have seen it." He handed it to her.

"I think so," she said.

"Here," Dr. Hopper indicated by pointing to the "Other Wishes" section, "he wrote that he would not wish to have artificial feeding. Perhaps he changed his mind?" Dr. Hopper looked back up at Helen.

"Yes, I think his mind did change," she said.

Dr. Hopper tilted his head and gave her a quizzical look. "Okay. If you're sure, then you would remember best." He paused. "And you are sure?"

She looked at the assemblage and nodded. She blinked and thought of bringing out the doctored directive that she had shown the ICU team. Then she realized that it was too similar to the one in Dr. Hopper's hand.

When Dr. Hopper finally left, Helen went back to the room, drew the curtain between Sean and the nearest patient. She nudged his body over, turning him to expose his back, and laid down behind him on this bed built for one. She pressed her chest against his back, propped her head up with her right arm, and grasped his waist with her left. She feels him press toward her. Only then, together with their eyes trained on the wall, could they admire her assemblage like he had her Rokeby in London all those years ago.

Now an hour has passed, maybe two, with them lying there. The breath hisses through his dry mouth, and she remembers him the way he used to be. Indistinct voices approach and recede behind the curtain.

Self-Portrait of Mr. E

Meanwhile, Sean Edgewater drifts through the eternal, nonaccruing present of his new pared-down life. Nothing is subtracted or added. Ghostly people come and go. They make clucking sounds. They come close to his body and touch him. A kindhearted gibberish comes from their mouths. He feels a sort of awe of the mystery of things; it is all so brilliant. Everything is so endlessly new and beautiful and like nothing else again. He wants to tell them but finds his dry mouth has no way to say it. He shifts his right arm a bit, but it is weak. He wants to pull the painful tube out of his nose, but he can't. Pain runs up his spine. The colors are bright and alive, and he wants to be with them, to keep them, but they hide from him. People come and go and cluck. Now, he is on his side and feels a hand on his waist. He feels love lying beside him, warm, and presses towards it. He looks at the familiar puzzling pictures on the wall, then feels love inside himself, too. He thinks enough is enough.

Editorial Note: The representation of the neurological state of consciousness of this patient was derived solely from the author's imagination. End-of-life issues are complex and should be discussed with healthcare providers.

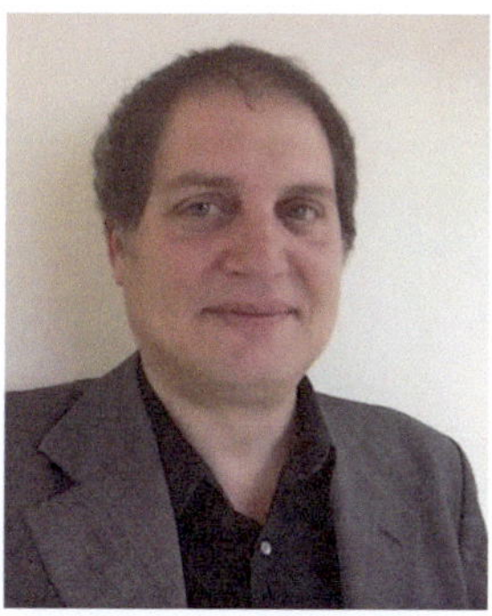

Dr. Steve Asch is a professor at Stanford and the Palo Alto VA. He is a general internist and palliative care physician. He is the author of many peer-reviewed articles and many fewer works of fiction.

14 The Birth Plan

Matthew Bucknor

We spent so long trying to pick a song. As if the sounds that he heard when he passed from the pressure and darkness into open air and light—as if the particular choice of key or cadence, harmony, or rhythm—that those few minutes of sound would define him and the scope of his aspirations and the extent of whatever small good change we might wish for him to bring to the world. I wanted Debussy, but Zoe laughed that straight back in my face. We settled on *Best Part,* a modern R&B classic, the slow burn of two soft voices longing for new love. Aside from the hospital and the obstetrician and the commitment to an epidural as early as seemed allowable, this was the only birth plan we had made.

Against the backdrop of this melody, I stare at my new son across the room, laying under the artificial heat of the infant warmer. Elijah. He stares back at me—I know he can't see me yet, but his deep brown eyes pour all over me. His limbs flail, but otherwise he is quiet. "A little too quiet," the nurse says, and so she places a small needle into his heel to check his blood sugar, to

First published in Intima: A Journal of Narrative Medicine

M. Bucknor (✉)
Department of Radiology and Biomedical Imaging, University of California San Francisco, San Francisco, CA, USA

J. Pien et al. (eds.), *Onward*,
https://doi.org/10.1007/978-3-032-15776-8_14

which he emits a piercing squeal and graceful arc of urine, which lands in her hair.

I know this is funny, and I want to laugh, but I can't laugh right now because I know what arterial blood looks like and I know the code words they're saying that mean, "it's not stopping," but Zoe doesn't know. She can't see or feel what is happening within and beneath her, and so, instead, I hold her gaze firmly, tears streaming down my face, and I say to her, "You did it. You're amazing. I love you so much." I say these words over and over, as if I can't think of anything else to say, which is true, because as these words fall out of my mouth, all I can otherwise think is *please don't leave me* and *I can't do this alone.* I feel as if I am being ripped clean in two.

Zoe closes her eyes. Her light olive skin is coated in beads of sweat, magnifying scattered brown freckles. Her darling Afro puff has collapsed under its own weight, flopped to one side of her head. *You are the most wondrous and beautiful thing I have ever seen*, I think. I turn the words over in my head. I am terrified to say them out loud because they sound deeply honest and tender; the kind of words you remember saying before someone close to you is lost. But the light panic at the foot of the bed is steady. And the blood dripping from the corner of one bedsheet is falling faster, like an IV line slowly opened. And so I turn back to Zoe's face and bring my lips close to her ear and I say, "You are the most wondrous and beautiful thing I have ever seen." She squeezes my fingers limply and centers my palm against her chest.

When we first checked into reception for labor and delivery, Zoe pleaded with me to tell the staff I was an oncologist. "Sweetie, I'm not sharing a room and I don't want to see a medical student at any point in the next month. So please be a darling and tell them you're a doctor and not your typical friendly Negro?" She said this with my favorite of her smiles—top teeth dominant, the small gap between central incisors on full display, lush ruddy bottom lip covering the rest. It took all my strength to deny her. But the sentiment felt too much like a threat, like fear under duress, which is not how I wanted our son to greet this world. Never mind the risk of doubt. So, I whispered, "Let's wait and see," and as luck would have it, there were only private rooms available and no medical students on the floor.

More nurses come into the room, gathering near my wife's feet, staring in the general vicinity of her groin. I know things are getting worse. I know that normally there wouldn't be this many people in the room, that there should just be the three of us, held together close under the spell of new life. Part of me wants to yell at them, "Do you know I'm a doctor?!" As if they are saving their compassion and skill for another set of patients. As if I have failed Zoe by not acquiescing to her earlier request. I know it defies logic, but I look back at her face, which has turned ashen, and all I can imagine is the color draining away until she is an alternating collage of blacks and whites, the color of newsprint, the color of the stories of new Black mothers dying that I can't seem to escape, the ones that make me cry into the crevices of my keyboard every single time.

The life continues to pour out of her. I am frozen, impotent. Wishful that, if I hold perfectly still, this moment could reverse itself. That this monster threatening to consume us might not see our small family of three in my stillness.

They are saying the placenta was "low-lying." They are pumping Zoe full of hormones meant to stop the bleeding. They are calling out her blood type—O positive. The delivering obstetrician presses firmly on Zoe's pelvis in a circular motion. With the other hand, she inserts a decompressed balloon into Zoe's bleeding womb and inflates the device. I check off each action in my head as if one misstep would require me to take over. Glistening suture and needle in a gloved hand, standing at the foot of the bed. *And then what?* I think. *And then what?* I grow more resolved in my stillness.

A circulating nurse brings Elijah to Zoe's chest. The look in the woman's eyes is severe—a look I can only read as: *enjoy this brief moment while you still have it, you will not have it for long.* Elijah's skin is a pale brown, paler than I imagined, and it occurs to me that he has not yet seen the sun. That he might not be held by his mother in the amber light of dawn, or blistering heat of midday, or soft glow of dusk. Zoe's eyes spring open as his weight settles into her. She takes his head filled with dark curly hair and presses his cheek against her breast. Her eyes dance all over his body. They recognize every single cell in an instant. She makes a noise that sounds at first like hysteria, then grows quiet, the soft coos intermittently drowned out by sniffling sobs and wet kisses: "He's so beautiful…Elijah, I love you…Elijah, thank you…"

Then, she turns to me and says, "Geoffrey, call my mother. Call her and tell her everyone's okay."

Zoe's mother, Michelle, had lived with us for two long weeks, a week before and after the due date. I knew better than to argue this arrangement. Her sister Katrina had lost a son the day he was born, and Michelle had always blamed her absence for the abbreviated life. As if some matriarchal spell was lacking in the minutes after birth, which might have prevented the tragedy. She would have waited even longer for Elijah but would have almost certainly lost her job.

I take my phone from my pocket. "There's no reception, Zo. I'll go out in a few minutes."

Zoe shakes her head dismissively and points to the door.

My eyes glance down toward the obstetrician, Dr. Kahn, who immediately holds my stare. I'm not sure if she is trying to tell me something. Trying to tell me not to go. I turn back to Zoe. "Baby, I think I should stay with you. I think it can wait."

"Geoffrey, please just call her real quick and come right back. Everything's okay."

I look again directly at Dr. Kahn. She is a smartly dressed, middle-aged woman in fitted purple scrubs, with round tortoise shell frames across her brow. She is not the obstetrician Zoe had seen throughout the pregnancy, but was on call covering the group. There is an inexplicable look of calm surrounding her, and I lean into that space. I'm not sure how to ask. I hold her eyes while I respond to Zoe, "I'm just a little worried baby, you're bleeding a little…"

"Worried?" the doctor snaps, with an ironic smile across her lips. "You can't be worried."

I look at her perplexed.

"Do I look worried?" she asks. She verifies first with Zoe, who shakes her head and smiles.

"Um, no, I don't think so."

"You neither." She stares firmly at me and punctuates the last syllable as if trying to hit me with a pair of forceps. Then she turns to Zoe: "Sweetie, you had some bleeding afterwards, but I think it's stopped. Everything looks stable. We're going to leave this balloon here for the first 24 h to make sure, but we should be able to take it out tomorrow. Don't worry." She glances at me again with that last word.

I look down at the sheets along the side of the bed, soaked in a light red hue. There's only stillness. Miraculous, wonderful stillness. I turn back to Zoe's face, which remains pale, but a slight hint of color has returned.

"Call. My. Mother."

***

I pace in circles outside the door to Zoe's room, holding my cellphone out like a metal detector in search of signal, but no luck. Briefly, I consider asking at the nurses' station but there are only faces buried in computer screens and I feel incapable of the small talk required to intrude. I walk quickly down the hallway and out of the maternity ward. My phone flickers between one and two bars of signal, but the call still won't go through.

Eventually, I take the elevators down to the first floor and exit the hospital. There is a thick, driving rain, and my shirt is drenched in seconds, but the phone call is brief. I tell Michelle that Zoe and Elijah are happy and healthy. I can't quite make out her blubbering response, except that she makes me promise to send pictures soon. She kisses the receiver repeatedly, and we both say goodbye in a fit of laughter. I hang up and yell nonsense words at the top of my lungs into dark gray San Francisco clouds. I laugh and cry and head back to the main entrance, then up the elevator to maternity.

When I buzz the ringer to be let in, at first, there is no response. I buzz again and hear a disembodied voice float through the speaker, "Can I help you, sir?"

I slide a few steps over to visualize the gatekeeper. She is a thin woman in pink scrubs, with short blond hair cropped beneath her ears. I'm guessing she's about my age, but it's unclear if she's a nurse or a medical assistant or a security guard. Her name tag reads, "Beth."

"Can I help you?" Beth asks.

"Yes, thanks. I need to get back to my wife, she just delivered." "What's the name?"

"Elijah."

She looks at me blankly. "Your wife's name."

"Sorry, Zoe Porter." "And you are?"

"Her husband…Geoffrey Martin."

"Mr. Martin, do you have a wrist band?" "No. What wrist band?"

"The matching wrist bands that the three of you are supposed to have. Where's yours?"

I look down forlornly at my naked wrist. "I don't know. She was bleeding, a lot was going on, I think they forgot. And then I went out to call her mom. Didn't you see me leave?" "No."

"Maybe someone else was here. Please could you just let me in? She had a postpartum hemorrhage, bleeding after the birth. I need to get back to her." I pray that I have said the words "postpartum hemorrhage" with enough clarity and confidence that she will be dissuaded from further inquiry.

"Give me one second, okay? Just need to check one thing."

I pace the few feet next to the door like a classic expectant father. I know Zoe and Elijah are fine—I'm pretty sure—but the minutes tick away, and I feel myself slowly unnerve. At first, it's only a slight quickening in my chest; breaths consumed in rapid succession, eyes unable to rest. But I can see the nursery across the hallway, and the indignation becomes more acute. *You should have told them*, I think.

I begin to press the buzzer every few seconds. It sounds like an abrasive rotary telephone. But there's not even the faintest response, not a hint of movement on the other side of the window. Then, I hit the steel door. It's thick, reinforced metal and makes no sound at all. I shift to the thin pane of glass next to the door and pound in raps of three. A few staff in the distance glance in my direction, puzzled, and then return to their respective work. I pound harder and harder until the knocking is audible, until the pain sears at the edge of my knuckles. I see Beth at the opposite end of the hallway, whispering into the ear of a security guard, but she makes no effort to move back toward the door.

Suddenly, I'm undone. I hit the glass harder still and waved frantically at Beth like we are old friends. I alternate punches with my hands, like a boxer working a body bag, my breath wincing with each blow, until thin streaks of blood run down my knuckles, and the glass begins to crack, then dent, and finally explodes into a small shimmering firework of tiny crystal splinters.

I survey my injured hand in disbelief.

Calmly, I reach through the broken glass and rotate the handle until the door slowly creaks inward. I stare at the ground, at the remnants of the broken window spread over brown linoleum. There is an eerie quiet on the unit, punctuated by occasional outbursts of maternal and fetal heart rate monitors. Countless sets of eyes are trained on me. I walk quickly into Zoe's room with my gaze cast downward.

Inside, everyone has left. It's just her and Elijah sleeping peacefully. And me. I walk to her and take our son from her arms and hold him up to the light. Then I climb into the bed and tuck Elijah between us. I remove my shirt so my chest is pressed directly against his back with his against hers—all skin to skin. I hold my phone up to the ceiling and take a selfie.

None of us smiles. Zoe asks me why my hands are bleeding, but I shush her and squeeze them both closer, while I wait for the others to come.

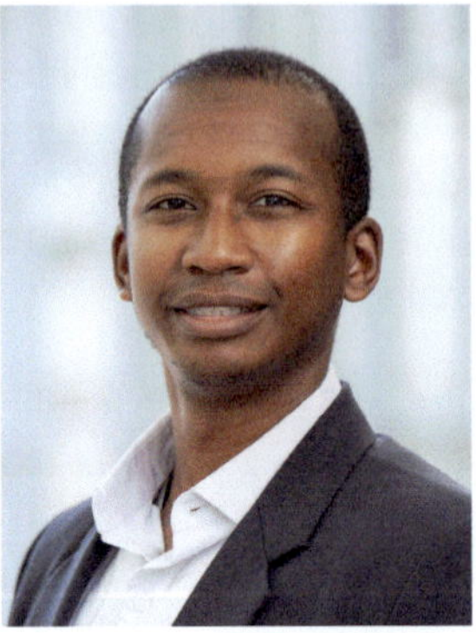

Dr. Matthew Bucknor is a Professor in Residence in the Musculoskeletal Imaging subspecialty section and the Associate Chair for Wellbeing and Professional Climate in the UCSF Department of Radiology and Biomedical Imaging. He is also the Executive Sponsor of Differences Matter, a UCSF School of Medicine multi-year initiative designed to support opportunity and belonging. He received his medical degree from Stanford School of Medicine and completed his four-year residency in Diagnostic Radiology at UCSF, followed by a clinical fellowship in Musculoskeletal Imaging and Intervention at Stanford Medical Center.

He is an Executive Board member of the Pegasus Physician Writers at Stanford.

The Medical Mystery of Ben Oco

15

Arjun S. Byju

Ben Oco regarded the pill bottle in his hand, lifting it to a pallid, incandescent light. Tears rolling down his cheeks, breath laden with alcohol, he twisted off the cap and shook the bottle's contents onto his palm. He wept as he tossed the 11 capsules into his mouth and gulped sloppily from his bottle of gin. The room, which had been spinning for more than half an hour, began to droop. Ben swiped at his wet eyes, wondering whether his vision was marred by the tears, the pills, or the booze. He thought maybe all of the above. Before he could reach his bedroom, he stumbled and fell face-first onto the floor.

First presented as "A 30-Year-Old Male with Idiopathic Hypotension and Tachycardia" at the Biannual Society for Medical Anthropology, Plenary Session on Ethnomedicine and Inert Pharmacopeia, Rochester, NY, 2019.

First published in the Pegasus Review

A. S. Byju (✉)
Department of Radiology, University of California Davis, Medical Center, Sacramento, CA, USA
e-mail: arjunsbyju@gmail.com

J. Pien et al. (eds.), *Onward*,
https://doi.org/10.1007/978-3-032-15776-8_15

The paramedics found Ben in this position, prone on his grandmother's Turkish rug.[1] Fifteen minutes later, he was in the Emergency Room with a blood pressure of 74/40 and a heart rate of 120. With the evidence hinting at attempted suicide, the clinical team forwent differential diagnosis and administered IV fluids and advanced life support. As the floor nurses began gastric lavage, an assiduous resident contacted Toxicology and Poison Control.

***

From the moment of Ben Oco's conception, he had been the most obliging of children. His mother, Philomena Oco (née Bloucher), and father, Tiberius Duryodhan Oco, recalled a remarkably painless delivery following what had been an even more comfortable gestation. Ben did not kick once the entire 9 months, nor did he beset his mother with an afternoon of lumbar pain. At exactly the 40th week, on the 280th day, Philomena had the fleeting thought that it would be a convenient time to have her child.

And so, he emerged. Seeming to desire to spare even the obstetrician the nuisance of providing a slap to the bottom, Ben Oco wailed on cue—softly, of course, and in the most mellifluous tone ever to coat the halls of St. Elizabeth's L&D floor.

Every person who met baby Ben agreed that he was the most pleasant child they had ever laid eyes on. In kindergarten, he shared his toys dutifully and stood statuesquely erect for each morning's recital of the Pledge. What some viewed as obsessive munificence and fastidious patriotism, his parents understood to be their son's cardinal trait: his willingness to please. Teachers, playmates, and even total strangers were enamored with Ben. He completed homework promptly, made every social engagement to

[1] A conscientious neighbor residing in the apartment below Ben's, after hearing an unceremonious thud around 9 pm, called 9-1-1. Mr. Maxwell Higglethorpe Lightfoot IV, a sophomore at Haverford College (Haverford, PA) and investment banking summer intern, claims to have had only one previous interaction with Mr. Oco. Three weekends before, Oco had knocked on the door of Mr. Lightfoot's apartment to politely ask that he and his squash teammates reduce the noise at their end-of-season party.

which he was extended an invitation, and affably played cards with his senescent grandparents each weekend at their retirement home.

While Philomena marveled at Ben's natural social grace and effortless popularity, Tiberius grew increasingly worried for his son. Ben's father, who had once studied Classics—with a significant emphasis on Greek tragedy—considered his boy's perpetual drive to do what others wanted a poignant *hamartia*. What would happen if thieves asked Ben to rob a bank for them? What kind of moral backbone could his son have if his behavior was so inherently impressionable?[2]

As time wore on, what Tiberius feared a fatal flaw proved to be Ben's greatest boon. At a college fraternity party, Ben once noticed a member of the men's lacrosse team making untoward advances on a female student. Despite overwhelming pressure to "mind his own business," he managed to whisk the girl back to her apartment, tuck her into bed, and return to the soirée in time to provide a stern reprimand to the young man in question. Unsatisfied with the bro's paltry apology, the next week Ben spearheaded a Title IX task force on the university's culture of sexual assault, eventually securing a campus-wide ban on Greek life.

Not wanting to leave a void in the partying ecosystem at his university, Ben created his own co-ed social organization, The Scene, which succeeded in eschewing both the traditionally toxic chauvinism of fraternities and the snobbish air of Final Clubs and Secret Societies.[3] Most bafflingly, Ben's crusade earned him no

[2]To this day, Tiberius Duryodhan Oco claims the ability to quote vast swaths of *Antigone* by-heart. Indeed, as his son deteriorated in the ICU, Tiberius could be heard lamenting, "Go then, if you must. But remember, no matter how foolish your deeds, those who love you will love you still." I looked up the phrase and found that it is, in fact, verbatim Sophocles.

[3]Of note, by the time Maxwell Higglethorpe Lightfoot IV (see footnote 1) attended university, The Scene had gained such national popularity that the young man would break with eight generations of family tradition and decline admission to the Frog and Sceptre—the college's oldest and otherwise most prestigious Eating Club—to partake in the decidedly nonexclusive debauchery of The Scene.

significant ire from former members of fraternities and sororities but only praise and abundant fist-bumps. As The Scene erupted in popularity, Ben was increasingly regarded as a somewhat Martin Luther-esque figure, responsible for reforming a salacious and decadent Pan-Hellenic system to its pristine and original purpose: the party.

Ben's unique talents also led him to career opportunities. Due to his knack for discovering what others really wanted, and not simply what they outwardly professed, he facilitated all manner of negotiations, settlements, and contracts, often between multinational corporations and litigants in class-action suits. His ability to please any and all parties led to his recruitment by the United Nations as a mediator during the Angolan Civil War,[4] and by the time he was 21, Ben had flown to Korea's DMZ at least three dozen times.

His novel gift was a sort of vicarious pliability; he yielded to demands that delegates themselves did not see meriting acquiescence, while never once conceding on principles. At the time of his suicide attempt, Ben was mastering both Hebrew and Arabic in anticipation of an unprecedented Palestine-Israel peace summit.

***

Even with such dazzling adventures, the most important thing to happen to Ben Oco was falling in love. Reed Sipson was a summer intern at the U.N. investigating reparations for descendants of the victims of the Thirty Years' War when she met Ben Oco.[5] They had struck up a friendship after quite literally bumping into each other in East River Park, where Ben had been absorbed in the

[4]Despite a purported commitment to impartiality, Ben was rumored to have held a particularly soft spot for the Front for the Liberation of the Enclave of Cabinda (FLEC), allegedly once dining with the separatist group's former leader, Henrique N'zita Tiago.

[5]For readers less familiar with their AP History: the conflict took place from 1618 to 1648 (hence the name) and involved an ensemble of Central European princely states. The war is generally considered to have started with the Defenestration of Prague (that is, the throwing out of a window) and roughly ended with a series of treaties known as the Peace of Westphalia.

terms of the Camp David Accords, and Reed was musing, chin to chest, on how to secure recompense from a long-defunct Holy Roman Empire.

Thus began an exciting courtship. Ben and Reed took frequent strolls along the river where they first met, made secret escapades into the World Health Organization HQ (where all the good snacks were kept), and freed a harbor seal from the New York Aquarium, driving it in an aqua-outfitted U-Haul truck to its home in the Puget Sound.

When the summer ended, Reed and Ben returned to their respective campuses to finish their senior years. For an entire 10 months, the couple communicated exclusively by post, Reed having a penchant for all things arcane (see her interest in seventeenth-century religious wars) and Ben having such an exceedingly pleasing nature to never demand an email or video call. Despite their anachronistic means of conversation, Ben and Reed's relationship blossomed during this year apart. After graduation, they moved together into a one-bedroom apartment.

To Ben, their relationship was perfect. Reed was compassionate and beautiful, and her idiosyncrasies and persuasions gave him something to which he could direct his powers of gratification. If Reed surmised that a proper gentleman ought to wear a hat, in the manner of every American president pre-JFK, Ben would don one. Once she commented that Ben had put on a bit of mid-section adiposity—completely understandable given the demands of his work. The next day, he joined a 24-h gym, and within 1 month, presented her with a pack of rippling abdominals. As the couple progressed from dating to engagement to marriage, Ben Oco found himself continuously challenged, rewarded, and ultimately fulfilled.

As in the rest of his life, Ben's unflagging desire to entertain the happiness of all around him verged on the extreme. To show his appreciation for Reed's cooking, he always ate whatever she prepared for him, even demanding second and third helpings. Growing suspicious, Reed once swapped salt for sugar in a chocolate chip cookie recipe. Happily, Ben scarfed the whole batch, rubbing his then chiseled stomach and burping contentedly.[6]

While Reed was initially offended (did her husband really care about her or did he just say "yes" to everything?), she came to realize that behind Ben's preternatural and inherent goodwill was a simple aim: for those around him to be happy, and to share in what they desired.

And this was not a bad thing. Ben supported Reed's career as she ascended the rungs of the Institute for Reparative Studies (IRS).[7] When it came to having children, Ben valued and respected her opinion, even though he desperately wanted to be a father. If they chose not to become parents, the Oco's would still have strong family ties and could be the most involved uncle and aunt to their niece.

In this way, Ben never rolled over as much as he moved the line in the sand. He reframed apparent dichotomies. He let both parties come away with a bigger slice of the pie. People who knew him were fond of mixing such metaphors.

Most importantly, to his wife, Ben was not ingratiating, just gracious. As Reed liked to joke with her friends, a sycophantic husband was even worse than an alcoholic one. Ben, as everyone could attest, was neither.

***

In one area, however, Ben's power to please failed him. As the years of marriage wore on, and the honeymoon became homeostasis, Ben struggled with the fact that no matter what he did, he could never free Reed from the cloud that had followed her since adolescence. He could make her laugh till she gasped for air, and he could make

[6]As readers might be aware, in certain Asian cultures—of which Ben was weakly extracted on the paternal side—it is considered not only polite, but extremely complimentary to a chef to belch boisterously after a meal. Ben had picked up this habit along with a handful of other culturally relativistic tics in his travels.

[7]The unfortunateness of the NGO's acronym was not lost on its employees, who viewed their task of making beneficiaries out of the wronged and otherwise indigent as diametrically opposed to that of Uncle Sam's extractive Revenue Service.

her smile for an entire afternoon, but the shadows always returned, and they laid upon her the weight of her entire lifetime.

Reed went days without eating. She cried everywhere and at random. So common was it for her to stay in bed until the afternoon that she would have lost her position at the IRS if not for Ben's frequent pleading with her boss. Still, there was nothing her husband could do, no task he could complete, to truly and fundamentally make her happy.

For years, Ben searched for an underlying problem, a cause for such inexplicable effects. Did Reed suffer from a profound lack of fulfillment? Or was her psyche tormented by abuse long repressed?

Ben goaded her to try all forms of remedies. Yoga, St. John's Wort, and "putting it into the right perspective" assuaged her sadness—but never cured it. Trips to Bali and stints of Japanese forest-bathing (*shinrin-yoku*) brought comfort, not bliss. Reed saw psychologists and psychiatrists, but also psychics and astrologers and even a Haitian *Houngan.*[8] By the time she was 29, Reed had tried every drug on the market: tricyclics, MAOIs, SSRIs, and the atypicals. She had done CBT and ECT. And she had completed three stints as an inpatient.

Of course, there were good days and good weeks—and even stretches of months during which Reed's profound sadness evaporated. But invariably it would return, sluggish at first, and then condensing, resolutely absorbing her once more.

Ben Oco was wracked by the realization that for the first time in his life, when it was more important than ever, he was incapable of making a situation better. The country's top scholar on mood disorders, whose consultation had been secured by Ben's eminent charm and goodwill, assured him that there was absolutely nothing he could *do* about the situation. Some things were simply a question of "chemical imbalance."

This fact Ben could not accept, and his attempts to fix his wife's situation, to be the mediator between her illness and her health, became increasingly desperate. He traveled to Peru, hiking 13 miles through the Andes to receive a rare crystal believed to

[8]A male priest in the Voudou tradition. The *Houngan's* female counterpart is known as a *Mambo.*

wield the healing power of the Incas. In a moment of despair and anger at her husband's inability to accept his own impotence, Reed threw the crystal into the garbage. Ben waded through the city's putrid landfill only to find that his wife would not accept the sludge-covered gem.

He bought her stuffed teddy bears, wrote sappy sonnets, and made her sweet potato gnocchi with hand-pressed Tuscan truffle oil. He even taught himself how to steer a sailboat with only celestial guidance to satisfy Reed's anachronistic interest in primitive navigation. Yet, Ben's wretched attempts at saving his wife from her own desolation hurt more than they helped. Reed started to believe that her husband endeavored in his silly way not because he wanted her to be happy, but to prove to himself, and the world, that he could make her so.

Thus, on May 11, 3 days after Ben turned 30, Reed struck up an affair with her chiropractor. A man in possession of an incredibly lucrative practice and a most vapid mind, Dr.[9] Barstone's preferred topics of discussion included the horrible hypocrisy of continental breakfast, the value of Bitcoin (and cryptocurrency in general), his heart rate, and a cruise he once took with an ex-girlfriend to Cancun.

At first, it pained Reed to engage in such fatuous conversation. Yet, as she returned home to find Ben's excessively earnest presents (like an original signed copy of the Mayflower Compact) waiting on the kitchen counter, the obscenity of her husband's overtures, the shamelessness of his attempts to cheer, eviscerated her even more than perfidy could. Lying in Dr. B's bed, his meaty hands against her cheek, Reed stared at the chiropractor's plasma TV—bought, she was told, at a devilish discount on Black

[9]"Doctor" was a title by which he insisted to be referred in all professional and nonprofessional situations. Ironically, it was Ben who first encouraged Reed to see this practitioner of vertebral subluxation in the hopes that some good, old-fashioned back cracking might snap her mind out of its catacomb of misery. As I have alluded to above, Ben was *very* desperate. *

* Your author, an unabashed allopath, has few scruples with "alternative medicine," as it is so often categorized, but a humane fellow ought to decry quackery when he sees it. Incan crystals and Haitian Voudou are one thing; skeletal skullduggery of the kind practiced by your run-of-the-mill-strip-mall Chiropractor is quite another.

Friday—and thought that maybe there was something more superior about modern entertainment and telecommunication. After all, writing letters really was so old-fashioned.

***

When Reed informed her husband about her affair, Ben Oco was characteristically calm. He listened quietly as Reed described the seriousness of her relationship with Dr. B. It had evidently moved quickly; Reed and the chiropractor were presently participating in couples tanning classes in anticipation of a trip to an all-inclusive resort in the Dominican Republic. They had already completed half of the melanoblastic sessions and had paid for the vacation in advance.[10] The relationship was steadfast, Ben was told. There was no hope, even for a charmer like himself, of dismantling it.

Here, Ben was confronted with a disheartening conclusion. First and foremost, he wanted to make Reed happy. Yet, Reed was supposedly happy with Dr. B. To please the woman he loved most in the world, a task at which he had been applying himself for the last 7 years, he would have to leave her to the consummate charlatan.

The syllogism of his mind dictated as such, so that very afternoon, Ben Oco decided to help Reed Sipson move in with the chiropractor. Before packing boxes of his wife's things, Ben contacted a fleet of auction houses; the pair had accumulated a great many knick-knacks in their years together, some of considerable historical and archaeological import. As Ben politely bartered with a purchasing officer from Sotheby's about vintage colonial-era contracts, Reed sat blankly on the sofa.

What she did not see was how Ben Oco, selfless as always, kept his grief and suffering to himself. After Reed moved in with Dr. B, Ben's downward spiral was precipitous and pitiable.[11] He

[10] A popular refrain at the time: "Couples who bronze together stay together." Later, an investigation by the Federal Trade Commission would reveal that much of the aggressively sentimental tanning industry advertising was funded by the American Dermatological Association.

[11] To be more medically and psychiatrically precise, I ought to describe this period in Ben's life as "acute decompensation." Terms like "downward spiral" are often unspecific and overused in lay publications, but in this case, I felt the phrase was apt: Ben really did decline like a swirling, vertiginous typhoon.

took up drinking, a hobby which he had never previously enjoyed, and ate only old-fashioned donuts for an entire month. His paunch flourished. He developed a mild form of agoraphobia, finding it difficult to leave his home for more than a few minutes at a time. He spent most of his time ambling from room to room, stroking the dust from old pictures, and watching cable news.

Every day, he would stare at his thin hands and cry, wondering why they were not dexterous enough at snapping and cracking like Dr. B's. Sometimes, he considered enrolling in a Doctor of Chiropractic program simply to see if he had what it took, but he always ended up ripping the application in a fit of shame.

He quit his job, the last role in which he was seriously applying himself. Halfway through a deal he was steering between House Republicans and Democrats, Ben stopped responding to texts, emails, or calls. His abrupt departure from one of the most challenging cases in his career contributed, in many ways, to a government shutdown. Ben accepted immense guilt for the furlough of thousands of federal employees, and silently sank into even deeper despair.

***

Ben saw his ex-wife not infrequently as she and the good doctor lived 20 min away in a neighboring suburb. Occasionally, he ran into Reed at the supermarket as he scurried to purchase canned tuna and packets of dried milk.

Still, he was surprised to find her one rainy morning, 5 months after they first parted ways, standing on his doorstep. She was chewing a piece of bright pink gum and gliding her thumb lazily on her smartphone. Reed informed Ben that she and Dr. B had just returned from their second Caribbean vacation. She had been *dying* to see him. It had been too long, she told Ben. She hoped he had been well.

She explained that she was stopping by to see if Ben had any of their old photos. If he did, she wanted very much to have them, if he could tolerate parting with such relics. Excitedly, Ben brought to the door a stack of pictures: the couple in Cambodia, climbing the Sleeping Giant in Kauai, posing with their rescued harbor seal. Reed smiled and thanked him.

Then, methodically, she pulled the backing from each frame, removing the pictures and matting. These she handed to Ben, who stood frozen. Reed looked up. Had he really expected her to keep the pictures? She merely wanted the frames—after all, they were vintage Gloucestershire oak. She tossed the empty wooden squares into the front seat of her car and, waving one final time, left forever.

That was when Ben Oco decided to kill himself. Despite all the people he had pleased and all the deals he had done, at that moment, Ben was as lonely and as displeased with himself as he ever would be.

He returned inside and started upon the gin. After an hour, he swung open the bathroom mirror and found Reed's old prescription bottles, left behind in the frenzy of moving. As he took a yellow bottle from the shelf, Ben wondered whether Reed still ordered her medications from the same pharmacy, or whether she had finally been cured, had found relief from her chemical disequilibrium.

***

Thus, I met Ben Oco, tachycardic and hypotensive, in the Emergency Room. He had a large hematoma on his forehead, from where he had fallen face-first, and his lips were powdered with the black of activated charcoal. He was obtunded and unresponsive except to painful stimuli.[12] His eyelids were barely able to conceal the waxen sclera of vision held back in its sockets. My residents had frantically awoken me; despite their earnest ministrations, Ben Oco was not recuperating. In fact, his hold on life, once vigorous and proud and gracious, was weakening by the minute.

[12]Meaning, no amount of shaking or pleading or snapping of fingers in ears could rouse the poor fellow. Stabbing a broken tongue depressor into the pad of his palm (the moderately painful stimulus) was the only way we could elicit a feeble whimper.

Sadly, there was little else I could do. In cases of suspected overdose, there is a standard protocol for emergency response, which my team had followed with exceeding readiness and care. Ben had been subjected, minutes after admission, to rapid sequence intubation. When his body began to seize and convulse, he was given benzodiazepines. To manage his precipitously low blood pressure, Ben's bed was tilted downward, and his circulatory system was infused with fluids. His stomach—once a powerful digester of modest acidity immune to bouts of reflux—was pumped of its former contents and plied with toxin-absorbing solutions.

Still, his condition did not improve. The team feared that the drugs had already reached his bloodstream and that Ben's life would soon come to a close. Inwardly, I feared something even worse: that Ben might live, but with permanent brain injury, an end more doleful than death itself.[13]

---

[13]In one memorably mordant lecture from my medical school days, a senior professor advised us against ever attempting to end our lives in this particular manner—the regrettably all too common concoction of prescription pills plus alcohol, he said, resulted in far more permanent brain injuries and vegetative states than eternal escapes from worldly suffering. Professor Reichburg also advised against the barrel-of-gun-to-bottom-of-chin approach. Apparently, the kick quite frequently caused an abrupt dorsiflexion of the head and thereby blasted off the would-be decedent's face, leaving him or her alive, albeit barely and severely mangled. He suggested that if ever the travails of medical education became insurmountable, we ought to stop by his office hours to inquire about the truly "best" method for final departure.

Unsurprisingly, these morsels of wisdom were not taken particularly well by the student body. The old professor's comments, which perhaps were accepted as jest by students of a bygone era, immediately elicited groans of discomfiture and even heckles from the lecture hall. Subsequently, the university received a storm of vituperative emails calling for Reichburg's prompt dismissal. Somehow the post-retirement-age professor stuck around for several more years and had a series of gaffes (or "generational misunderstandings" depending on whose opinion you polled) Eg: During a lecture about dietary sodium and water retention, Prof R. commented that he frequently advised borderline hypertensive patients against eating "ethnic foods" as they could, with their heightened salt content, contribute to an edematous episode.

Nevertheless, based on my 25 years of experience as an attending physician in the ER at a major urban hospital, I must admit that the codger's "advice" on suicide was largely accurate, if not somewhat gauche and offensive.

As the minutes wore on, Ben's chest rose ever more slowly. We watched helplessly as his ALT and AST skyrocketed, and his blood became unprecedentedly replete with urea and creatinine. His liver and kidneys, the twin powerhouses of toxin elimination, were shutting down. I barked at a supercilious medical student, scribbling furiously in a spiral notebook. Calculations of glomerular filtration could wait. So too could the EMR and the billing codes. Here, before our very eyes, was a man departing the world of the living, dying despite the most advanced biomedical technology humankind had to offer. It was a rare moment to behold, a moment deserving of respect.

And then, without even a shudder, Ben's electrocardiogram flat-lined. His heart had stopped.

As my team stood stoically silent, a third-year resident, Kalverina Machechnikova, flew into the room, panting and grasping at a pink sheet of paper. A member of the shift that first admitted Ben, Kalverina had held on to the pill bottle used in his suicide. She had looked up its prescription ID number and found that it was part of a Phase III, double-blind trial. A novel neurotransmitter inhibitor almost ready for market.

Wanting to learn how to counter the drug's toxicity, she called its manufacturer. To her immense surprise, she learned that the individual for whom the prescription had been written, one Reed Sipson, was assigned to the placebo arm of the trial. That is, the pills which Reed had been taking for 6 months prior to her divorce, and which her ex-husband had swallowed in one gigantic gulp, had consisted of nothing more than sugar and cellulose.

Kalverina held up the fax from the FDA's clinical trial manager, waving it around her head. The evidence was on the paper. The man lying at the center of the hospital room had not ingested anything more dangerous than a mildly sweetened iced tea.

Immediately, the EKG machine started to sound. Ben's heart erupted in a flutter of staccato beats. The monitors revealed his blood pressure creeping back to normal, his liver and kidney function accelerating at a heady pace. Slowly at first, his body began to wriggle and then, within minutes, he opened his eyes and looked around the room. The physicians, nurses, and technicians, who moments before were bowing heads and crossing chests, stood with their mouths irreverently agape. Within half an hour, drips removed, gown strewn mercilessly aside, Ben Oco stood up and walked out of the hospital.

Since then, according to most accounts, Ben has lived a largely unremarkable life. After his near-death, he seems to have lost the powers to solve and placate that had previously defined him. From what I have been told, the man is now much less impressionable and rarely, if ever, willing to please.

After quitting his international mediation practice, Ben now earns a modest living as a claims adjuster for a motorcycle insurance agency. In this capacity, he is reviled by victims of vehicular collisions; however, in stark contrast to his former self, Ben seems to care little about his clients or his reputation. Neighbors regard him as a cantankerous yet immaculate gardener.

I have had no interactions with Ben Oco since his dramatic stint in my hospital, although I think about his case often. Every few months, I search his name in our medical record database, hoping, selfishly, that he has been admitted again. Despite treatment for benign nasal polyps two months ago, he remains, to the best of my knowledge, in completely good health.[14]

***

[14]What is described in this report is not wholly without precedent. The medical literature details many cases in which patients have reported adverse effects from the consumption of non-active drugs. These negative placebos (or so-called nocebo effects) have been documented frequently in the reporting of side effects. For example, many patients—later revealed to have been taking a placebo—have complained of migraines, muscle aches, nausea, and irritability after prescription of a new drug. The effects can be more than psychological. Patients have presented with rashes, fevers, weight fluctuations, changes to blood sugar, aberrant lipid profiles, and reduced cardiac output. It appears that harmful physiology can manifest simply because one believes oneself to be consuming a harmful substance.

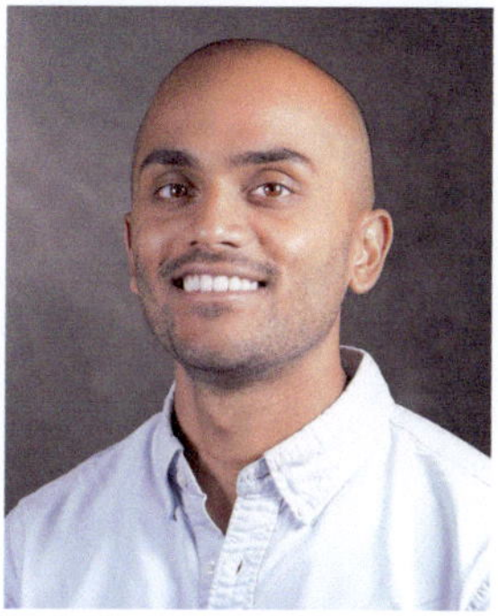

Arjun S. Byju is a writer and radiology resident at UC Davis Medical Center, and a graduate of Albert Einstein College of Medicine and Harvard College. His work has appeared in the *Los Angeles Review of Books*, the *New Republic*, *Current Affairs*, and *Natural History*, among others.

A Boundaried Love

16

Jennifer Pien

Elizabeth leaned towards me. "Kinsley is eating again."

Four words, but they might as well have been a torrent, because when she said them, something within my friend shifted, the lines on her brow easing. A storm's ending. It was the relieved exhalation of a breath held too long.

Elizabeth and I shared many things. A profession, a heritage, the joys and burdens of motherhood. Like myself, Elizabeth was a physician. But where I provided for those with heart issues, she worked as a rehabilitation doctor. An expert on mending the body after traumatic injury or guiding it through chronic debilitating conditions. In addition to our shared background in medicine, both our families were geographically disjointed—a scatterplot of relatives rimming the Pacific Ocean.

We met at a Starbucks, one with a smattering of metal chairs and tables pushed against each other. A kind couple asked if we were alright. Elizabeth's exhaustion and joy colored our ordinary. Not only was her teenage daughter eating again, but their relationship was stronger than ever. Despite her joy, or perhaps because of it, I could not help but remember our first meeting.

J. Pien (✉)
Department of Psychiatry and Behavioral Sciences, Stanford University School of Medicine, Stanford, CA, USA

J. Pien et al. (eds.), *Onward*,
https://doi.org/10.1007/978-3-032-15776-8_16

It was early December 2019. We walked together along the rolling knolls of Byxbee Park under overcast skies. Foamy waters marked the bay. We had connected over a shared patient and made commitments to develop a friendship. Elizabeth was grey, then, a shadow of the blazing woman I would share tears with a year later. We walked together and told our stories, marveling at the similarities. I listened as she confessed the helplessness she felt in the face of Kinsley's health crisis. "My love for my daughter is my shelter from the storm," she said. "What am I supposed to do when she becomes the storm?"

I thought about a sailor's terror when an anchor line snaps, or a beacon is snuffed, the moment of realization that events have been ripped beyond control. Kinsley was no stranger to that fear. Neither was Elizabeth. In fact, as one who has known asthma her entire life, she was well-versed in it.

A few months earlier, Elizabeth told me her 12-year-old's asthma had suddenly exacerbated. Kinsley was prescribed oral steroid treatment and soon recovered her breath. However, through the fall and winter, through the distractions of daily life, Kinsley began to change. Her appetite gradually lessened, she began to skip meals. Once a hearty omnivore, she developed specific, rigid tastes that excluded all comfort foods, as if eating rich or flavorful meals was somehow unbearably painful. At the same time, she continued to endure the endless and sometimes tedious changes that go hand-in-hand with the transformation to adulthood. A physician, Elizabeth was on alert for alterations signaling a shift from youth to adulthood. However, winter holidays, visiting in-laws, and preoccupations with the milestones and rigors of clinical work and school deadlines obscured her attentiveness. So that when the new year began, her child had withdrawn, her brightness dulled, her moods shifted. Were these the quintessential teen changes that haunt our culture, or was the increasing weight loss and food selectivity a harbinger of one of a mother's greatest fears—an adolescent onset of an eating disorder?

A new spring arrived. Protests blazed in Thailand. Elizabeth's in-laws fled the turmoil and merged with her family, trapped here without health insurance once the pandemic hit. Prone to fainting spells, falls, and other vague concerns, they were not entirely frail but nonetheless claimed the majority of her attention. Disorder upended her life. Amid the focus on her elders, she missed the insidious transition of Kinsley's worsening symptoms.

The symptoms spread. Homework assignments went uncompleted—Kinsley lacked the energy to focus. Once full of life and vibrancy, her moods soured. When she could no longer stand in the shower without assistance, Elizabeth turned in panic to a pediatrician. But it is easy to forget how terrifyingly like animals our children can sometimes be, unspeaking, without the typical somatic signaling that adult bodies are used to conveying and receiving.

"I'm a doctor…all our friends are doctors! And still, we were unable to find a specific diagnosis," she said to me at one of our meetings. A thick kind of fear clogged her gaze and hastened her breathing. I shifted forward. Even physicians have their moments of uncertainty and fear. I was not a specialist in eating disorders, but I could listen. "I had to reach out for help," she continued.

Lana, an adolescent medicine physician who spent every Thanksgiving with Elizabeth's family, held her hand through every step of Kinsley's illness, providing love and compassion to pull their family out of despair. "And of course, it was more than just Lana."

At first, Elizabeth's ability to so readily and easily reach out to others baffled me. I could not imagine doing the same. But I was going through my own struggles.

On the cusp of the pandemic, a guilt began to overwhelm me. It began as a scarcity of emotional capital, a perceived inability to meet the social needs of the various communities in which I was involved. All these states of motherhood, being a physician, etc., had their own social obligations and needed to be allotted portions of my energy. My emotional capital had been leached away by so many sources that it had run dry. The taxation of extroversion grew with no end in sight. But the majority narrative, from blue zone to loneliness studies to Hollywood, had, over the course of my life, taught me a painful lie, had reinforced the necessity of relentless extroversion and socialization as an essential component to happiness. Networking, PTA Fundraising events, work meetings, endless birthday brunches, baby showers, bouncy house kid parties, social media—had overtaken my life. The purported formula for happiness was clear.

Never be alone.

I was certainly not alone. Far from it. But I was also far from happy. A fog had settled over the edges of my life, a listlessness that pervaded every interaction I forced myself to endure throughout the day. The fog thickened, became a barrier that needed to be waded through, a shield that distanced me emotionally from the ones that I should have been closest to—my family and loved ones. The world was too busy, and too close around me, and I was at a loss for what to do, having exhausted all resources available simply to survive.

One evening, Elizabeth confided in me that she felt her social duties and interactions pulled her away from her daughter, that her preoccupation with satisfying the desires of others had caused her to miss what was happening to her daughter. "I was unhappy," she told me. "And then, when Kinsley became increasingly ill, I was afraid." But for both of us, at the height of our slowly rising panic, our emotional exhaustion, an unlikely and terrible savior appeared.

During the pandemic, many of the elders in my own family fell ill. My husband and I were suddenly tasked with the medical shepherding of extended family, of supporting relatives who, back in China, found themselves in dire straits. We WhatsApped, Lined, and WeChatted, scrolled through inscrutable medical records, connected with a sprawling network of physicians and colleagues and somehow made do. But what was stressful was also a refuge at times. Free of the constraints of social obligations, my fog lifted. I found new attention and time for my children and husband, for the passions that keep me vital and alive. Meanwhile, Elizabeth found herself with the same strange recalibration. She invested her newly claimed time in caring for her daughter.

Proust is infamous for his prolonged bouts of illness. It was only his health that forcibly removed the writer from his beloved dinner parties, thus giving him the time and reservoir of energy to write. He needed to be saved from himself. It took a devastating pandemic to save us both.

Early in the health crisis, Elizabeth maintained stringent caution; her uncertainty about the degree of spread or morbidity associated with COVID-19 led her to keep Kinsley at home, despite the urging of many doctors and friends, including Lana, to hospitalize her. With Lana's help, Elizabeth and her husband became all things adolescent medicine and devised a refeeding program at home. After nearly 6 months of battling this, when Kinsley told them that eating was too painful, that she would rather die than work through hour after hour of forced eating, their family of four held each other and cried.

Refeeding is neither a gentle nor an easy process. It is more like stopping a runaway train. The body, in its efforts towards self-preservation in the face of reduced calories, shuts itself down. It was Elizabeth's job to slow the train and then, with agonizing resilience, reverse its direction. Slowly, Kinsley's body would receive the signals it needed to return to life, banishing the atrophy of her appetite and reviving a nearly defunct gastrointestinal system.

Time passed. A diagnosis continued to elude them. Elizabeth faced difficult questions, quagmired in a lack of actionable knowledge. Was Kinsley evidencing, if not a psychiatric disorder, an organic disorder that plagued atopic children like herself? Eosinophilic esophagitis was a possible diagnosis. Should she be started on a regimen of steroids—the most common treatment? Elizabeth forged her way through the barriers imposed by the pandemic and managed to secure time with a pediatric gastroenterologist. She offered a possible diagnosis, one she saw frequently in post viral, post steroid patients. Gastritis. An inflammation so severe that children will stop eating, all the while evidencing no pain, no discomfort, no signaling. They simply stop eating.

Were the oral steroids that allowed Kinsley to breathe the very thing that prohibited her from eating? It seemed like a terrible irony, and in the meantime, her asthma continued to exacerbate as she grew weaker. She needed a new course of oral steroids; she needed to breathe, but the risk of administering them was immense. The steroids might treat the possible EOE Gastritis (the pandemic shut down access to EGD diagnostics) as well as Kinsley's asthma. But they might also radically increase the severity of a possible gastritis. Elizabeth told me her nights were fraught with shame, fear, and impotence—after all, what kind of parent fails to provide for their children's most basic imperatives? To breathe. To eat. To live.

Bite by bite, accompanied by cruel sips of Boost and spoonfuls of avocado oil that left Kinsley gagging, Elizabeth waded forward through the storm. The runaway train showed no sign of stopping, and the specter of gastric tubes, hospitalization, perhaps even Kinsley's death, awaited her failure to reverse it. But Elizabeth was a physiotherapist, well-versed in treating and preventing physical illness, and most importantly, being with patients as they weather their suffering: as a mother, she laid her daughter's head in her lap, soothed her, translated what her doctors were saying, and modified their intimidating directives to be more palatable. Held her as her daughter shared memes and Spotify songs that could express how tormented she was. As a physician, she had to feed and sustain Kinsley not only physically but emotionally. To dedicate herself solely to this task, Elizabeth needed isolation as much as she needed the help of others.

The story Elizabeth told me is one that goes against the grain, that it was not the elimination of solitude but rather the protection of it that allowed Elizabeth to chart a path through the challenges of not only her daughter's illness, but also the obstacles that exhausted her throughout her life. It was the pairing of deliberate isolation with tactical interactions with dear friends and community that allowed her survival. Freed from commutes and endless social compulsions, Elizabeth could focus her energy on something vital. The hecticness, the loudness, and the busyness of social obligations were eviscerated, burnt to the ground. Out of the ashes rose something stronger—the core relationships transformed into something unbreakable.

It is no coincidence that Woolf encouraged women to find "a room of one's own" or that Marcus Aurelius often retreated to what he named his "inner citadel." There are those, like Li Bai or Mahler, who withdrew to lakes and secret habitations embedded in nature, but most of us must carve out these havens within the existing constructs of our lives. As John Cowper Powery says in his Philosophy of Solitude, we must master the art of creating for ourselves a continuity of great happiness, in defiance of our world. But paradoxically, this solitude must be built on caring for and being responsible to a greater community, or we risk losing the equanimity that must accompany these times for reflection.

Elizabeth told me at the beginning that her love for her daughter was her shelter from the storm. But I believe that it was this quietude of the self, this solitude, that yielded the true shelter, and within it, a path back to her daughter.

Now, more than a year later, the lockdown over but still bearing masks, we sit on these off-kilter coffee shop chairs, and she tells me that her daughter has all but fully recovered from her gastritis, that her joy for life and her vitality have returned in full force. Oreos overflow their snack drawer. A smorgasbord of teen food horrors runs rampant through the home: In and Out. Pizza. Chick-fil-A. Milkshakes and a never-ending stream of boba tea. She tells me that the day Kinsley asked for khao tom, she wept and then ordered endless plates of noodles and rice.

There is something she says that I keep for myself, for the times when the fog returns, when my emotional capital is worn to shreds. "I will protect my choice for solitude, the time we must spend with ourselves and our intimates. A boundaried love." She smiles when she says it, and I cannot help but admire her newfound strength, the will behind each word.

We share a pastry. The storms of life rage on, but neither of us is lost. Together, and alone, we all find our way.

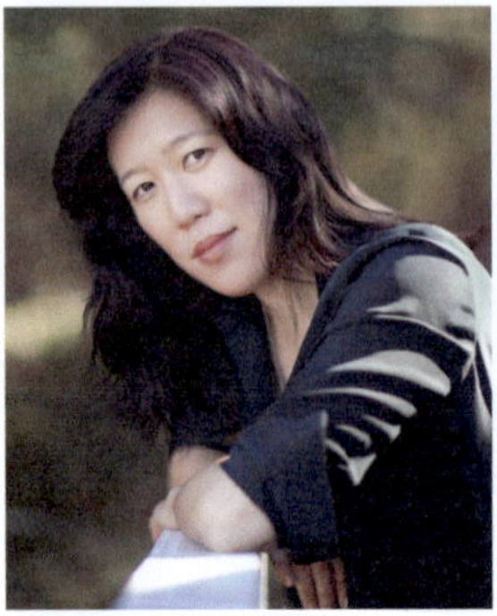

Jennifer Pien is a Clinical Associate Professor through the Department of Psychiatry at Stanford University. She is the Director of The Pegasus Physician Writers and is founding faculty for the Oxford Review of Books x Stanford Collaboration. She also serves on the Advisory Boards for The Bellevue Literary Press and the Stanford School of Medicine Medical Humanities Fellowship. Represented by Lisa Grubka of United Talent Agency for her fiction and Amy Collins of Talcott Notch for her nonfiction, Jennifer's upcoming book, Healing the Healers, is set to be published by Johns Hopkins University Press.

How to Deal with Charon 17

Brian Smith

How to Deal with Charon[1]

At first, you don't even try. Trying would mean acknowledging him. Instead, you focus on her and what her doctor is saying. There's whining in your ears. It could be your tinnitus or it could be your body protecting you from what's being said. Either way, it's so loud that you know it can't be a nightmare because you don't wake up. Something's closing in, and you're frozen in darkness, paralyzed, helpless. The doctor says, "It's cancer."

That's when the water announces Charon's arrival. Frigid, brackish, it gushes into the room. Your socks are soaked, but nobody wants to talk about it. The oncologist is probably used to the feeling, but it is new to you. The smell of rotting seaweed. A

[1] In Greek mythology, Charon is the ferryman whose duty it was to help people cross over the River Styx and enter the afterlife.

B. Smith (✉)
Department of Medicine, Stanford University School of Medicine, Stanford, CA, USA
e-mail: bsmith19@stanford.edu

J. Pien et al. (eds.), *Onward*,
https://doi.org/10.1007/978-3-032-15776-8_17

figurehead crosses the threshold: a tentacle holding a lantern. Everyone's been dancing around it, but the doctor finally broaches the subject. They explain the 5-year survival rate, and the ferryman glides in.

As you walk out of the clinic, she asks you to slow down. "Stop pulling my arm. What's the rush?" She hears a siren a few blocks down the road and nods, smiling as if letting you in on a joke. "They've found me, haven't they? Well, if this is the end, I won't go down without a fight." You smile and laugh, ushering her onward as you glance over your shoulder.

How do you deal with Charon? When you see him, you give him the finger.

You're past ignoring him because he shows up too often. When your cousin dies of a heart attack, the ferryman delivers the funeral invitation. You watch him check the pulse of the homeless man outside Safeway. He mans the desk at the infusion center and nods at her as she walks past. She nods back, and you wonder how she can be courteous to that asshole. When you see him, you swear. When she sees him, she sighs and waves. You don't understand their relationship, but you're not supposed to. She says they have a "mutual understanding," whatever that means. You'd rather stay positive and hope so hard that you manifest a world where he doesn't exist.

As the number of treatment cycles grows, you complain about the process and the waiting and the uncertainty and Charon. She glares at you and says, "Wow, I'm sorry, this must be so hard for you," and that shuts you up.

And then the bastard Freddy Krugers you, showing up in your nightmares. But at least here you can shout and scream and slash at him without making her cry.

How do you deal with Charon? Maybe it starts with looking in his eyes.

Meet his stare, even though it floods your veins with ice water and acid. You want to look away and pretend he does not exist, and she knows this. "I get that you don't want to talk about it," she says, "but we have to be prepared for the worst. I don't want to be the villain here," she says, "but do you really want to be the dick that argues with a cancer patient?"

So, she sits you down, and as she talks, it happens again—the water, your socks, his boat, him. You say that this is a private discussion, that you didn't agree to this threesome, but she says it's what she wants. On the same pad that she used to list groceries, she now lists her treatment options. She gets partway through before her hands are shaking too much. She turns to Charon and screams, "Why is this happening to me?" He doesn't reply. In between sobs, she asks, "What will give me more time?" He stays silent. You pick up the pen and continue her list.

You both sleep badly. At some point, she whispers, "Is this my fault?" and you both lie there, feeling the heft of the question press you into the mattress. And then you hear him move. You didn't know he was even there, so you lunge at him but fall through him. You land on the floor and spin, ready for another try, but you freeze. He is sitting on the bed, and they are looking at each other. He takes her hand and shakes his head.

You don't like it, but you let him stay. She says it's better than pretending he's not there.

Now, when you get home from work, sometimes you see the two of them sitting at the kitchen table. They're not friends, but she doesn't flinch when she looks at him anymore.

On your anniversary, she decides you're not going to bring him. Tickets to Hawaii aren't cheap. You ask her doctors to help, and they say they can make it happen. She takes potent meds to suffocate her nausea, her vomiting, her pain—the canaries that warn you he's coming. She asks you to find a less violent metaphor. You tell her you will but forget.

For a while, the afterglow of the islands keeps you warm, and Charon is only a memory.

He returns when her oncologists keep talking about treatments but stop talking about cures.

And then you get a call from the police that there's been an accident. You almost ask if Charon met her there but before you do they tell you where she is, which hospital, and you're out the door and driving 30 over because you're racing him and his fucking ferry and you wish your eyes had wipers too and you sprint in without locking your car and you find her room and she's there and he's not.

And then you can breathe.

She explains what the doctors told her, that she'd probably crashed because of a seizure. She says they already did a brain scan, and it had shown that it's spread there, too, invading that sacred temple. She uses a quiet, calm voice. You can tell she's trying to protect you. In your head, you see an hourglass, and you frantically try to block the fall of the sand, but it keeps slipping between your fingers.

Before the surgery, she kisses your hand. Some of her lipstick stays. You don't wash that hand until she's discharged home.

More and more, she pushes to talk about crossing the river. She starts saying "when" instead of "if." You still don't want to, but she's not going down without a fight, and it's not your call to make. She says it's not what is on the other side that she fears, but the crossing. "I wonder if Dylan Thomas changed his tune," she muses, "when he was dying. Raging against the dying of the light sounds like a lot of work. And pain. Do not go gentle into that good night?" she says, "Do not tempt me with a good time, Dylan."

They're together all the time now, and she looks more comfortable with him. So, you are not surprised when she says, "I don't want to fight it anymore." The palliative care referral is already placed. She makes her appointment.

Off of treatment, she smiles more. She sits a little straighter, as if a weight's been taken off. You look closer and realize Charon is helping her float, the water around him rising and cradling her. Something inside of you melts. You look at Charon. For the first time, you hate him *and* you don't.

She hands you a letter. "Don't read this until after," she says. "We wrote it together when I realized he would be the inevitable co-author of my life's last chapter. I waited to give it to you until I was sure you saw that, too."

And then, when it's time, this is how you deal with Charon:

You squeeze her hand and whisper, "I love you," kissing her forehead one more time. You beckon him closer and say, to both of them, "I'll see you again someday."

You place her hand gently in his.

You look him in the eyes and say, "Take care of her." He looks her in the eyes and nods.

He says, "I will."

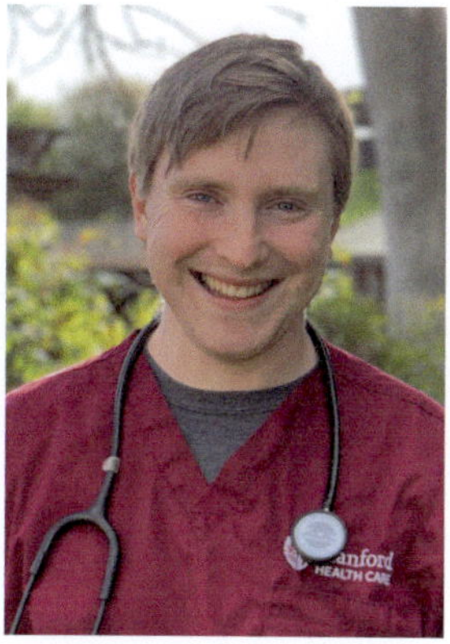

Brian Smith (he/him) is a medical student at the Stanford University School of Medicine. Before medical school, he worked as an oncology scribe. He considers working with oncology patients, their families, and their healthcare teams one of the greatest honors of his life. He is deeply involved in the medical humanities, and you can find his narrative medicine poetry, prose, and visual arts in over 20 academic journals, such as *Anesthesiology*, *Annals of Internal Medicine*, and *JAMA Oncology*. He finds healing, reflection, and hope in storytelling and hopes others will, too.

Index

J. Pien et al. (eds.), *Onward*,
https://doi.org/10.1007/978-3-032-15776-8

MIX
Papier aus verantwortungsvollen Quellen
Paper from responsible sources
FSC® C105338

If you have any concerns about our products,
you can contact us on
ProductSafety@springernature.com

In case Publisher is established outside the EU,
the EU authorized representative is:
Springer Nature Customer Service Center GmbH
Europaplatz 3, 69115 Heidelberg, Germany

Printed by Libri Plureos GmbH
in Hamburg, Germany